everyBODYmatters!

... including you(rs)

Simple Ways To
Improve Your HEALTH

Dr. Trishul Vadi
BOst, MChiro, PG Cert HE
Osteopath and Doctor of Chiropractic

ISBN: 9798494188052

DISCLAIMER

The book is for informational purposes only. Neither the publisher nor the author is engaged in rendering professional advice or services to the individual reader. The ideas, procedures and suggestions contained in this book are not intended as a substitute for consulting with your health professional. All matters regarding your health require professional supervision. Neither the author nor the publisher shall be liable or responsible for any loss or damage allegedly arising from any information or suggestion in this book.

While the author has made every effort to provide accurate information at the time of publication, neither the publisher nor the author assumes any responsibility for errors or for changes that occur after publication. Further, the publisher does not have any control over and does not assume any responsibility for author or third-party websites or their content.

DEDICATION

Dedicated to all who have entered our “home” – thank you for your trust in us!

ACKNOWLEDGMENTS

To our parents - Asha, Prafulla, Vijay and Anup, who without, not only would I literally not be here, but also, not be able to reach my true potential to impact the lives of others. You continue to inspire me to make you proud.

Komal, my wife, I cannot imagine sharing the front seat of this rollercoaster of life with anyone else by my side.

To our children, I will love you more than you will ever know. I do it all for you.

To all AVID "Family" – past and present – your shared passion & enthusiasm have helped make my vision a reality, to create a better world, long may this continue!

To all of our Guests, we would not be where we are, without you – thank you for letting us be a part of your journey of life!

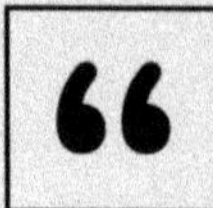

I started off with severe pain on the lower back, with just a few sessions I could start to notice a difference. Simple things like going to make a cup of tea became normal to life, whereas before it could take me a while to get to the kettle and would be a painful experience.

AVID Clinic has also helped me with my mental health. The staff are super friendly and are always there to listen, also I have confidence that if the pain starts to come back they can get back to normal. Coming to AVID has been one of the best decisions I've made and would 100% recommend anyone that suffers with back pain to give them a try.

Leigh McDonald

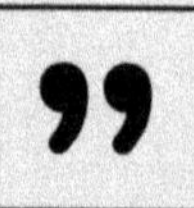

CONTENTS

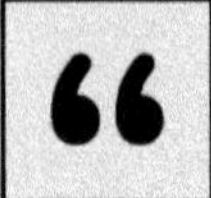

I went to see Trishul to help with some discomfort in my back. I'm now a couple of months into a treatment programme and feeling noticeably better. This isn't somewhere that will promise a miraculous result after one visit but will work with you to get things to where they should be over time in a realistic way.

Staff are all fantastically friendly, happy to have children visit with you (helpful in school holidays!) and it's a very personal service. I dithered about making the initial appointment for a long time, partly because there wasn't acute pain, but I shouldn't have - would highly recommend!

Ellen Migo

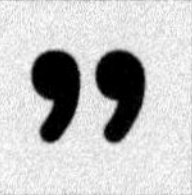

FOREWORD

Health is a spectrum.

The reason for our success over the years is based on a particular set of principles. The COVID-19 Pandemic has been the ultimate test to date of these principles. In this book I share how these sets of principles have stood the test of time and more importantly how you too can live the life you were meant to live without your health limiting you in any way.

Many enter our doors in pain and dysfunction, living their lives in a dimmed and disconnected state. It is our goal to use the very best techniques to reconnect your body to itself.

A reduction in pain and restoration of optimal function is, however, just the beginning. Health "is not merely the absence of disease" or pain; but rather living in a state of healing yourself, and this is our purpose:

To INSPIRE you to actively make positive changes to your life; physically, mentally and socially

To SERVE you with the highest quality, cutting edge, evidence-based care to give you the best possible results.

To GROW your expression of life, to reconnect your body and elevate your being.

Welcome to AVID where *everyBODYmatters*!

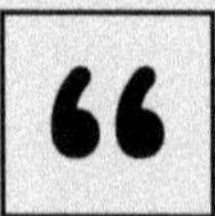

I began attending AVID Clinic due to me suffering from terrible back, neck and headaches which made sleeping and most normal daily activities really difficult. The pain in my neck and head started from working from home over a long period of time, however, the back pain had been ongoing for over 13 years during my pregnancy with my son.

AVID Clinic is such a lovely and relaxing environment to attend with very friendly and attentive staff. Trishul, the practitioner who helped me always explains what he is doing, how my body is adjusting and what the next steps are so I never feel worried or out of the loop. I feel really looked after attending this Clinic and I am quickly getting better thanks to Trishul and I am feeling stronger than I have done for years.

I travel quite a way to see Trishul but I am so happy that by chance, I saw Trishul's Instagram with his great work when I needed his care.

Natalie McNeish

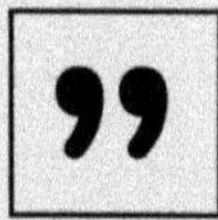

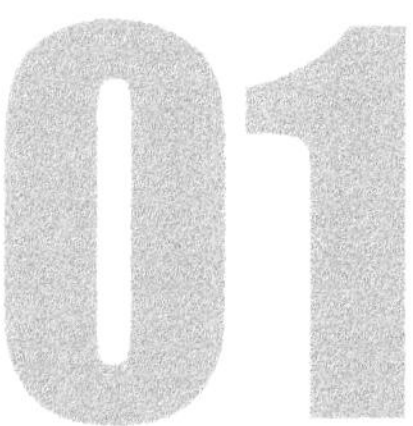

THE SICKNESS IN MODERN HEALTHCARE

"I think the biggest problem with healthcare today is not its cost – which is a big problem – but for all that money, it's not an expression of our humanity."
~Jonathan Bush

"Government doesn't solve problems—it subsidizes them."
~Ronald Reagan

I am student that had been recently suffering with a migraines, tinnitus, neck and back issues all spanning from the same time. I was very concerned as to what was causing this as for the most part I was very healthy. I started to look online with these symptoms to see if there was any link and it turned out there was a fair amount of people who had shared similar experiences as me and a common method they used to solve their issues was to see a chiropractor. After this I looked online to find which was the best chiropractor for me. The best one I found was AVID due to their well designed website, informative videos and the diverse services they offered. I booked straight away and was able to get an appointment very quickly. Upon going there, the staff were very lovely and made me feel reassured about the process. After the initials assessment they were able to identify the root of my problems and put me on a treatment plan which has been very successful and alleviated my issues drastically.

Josiah

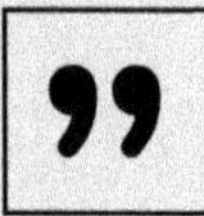

The biggest problems in the modern healthcare system throughout the world are the same: high costs, poor results, frequent medical errors, and patient dissatisfaction.[1] Simultaneously, we face a global epidemic of obesity and chronic disease. For example, cardiovascular disease, cancers, dementia and Alzheimer disease were the leading causes of deaths in the UK in 2018.[2]

The structure and function of the modern healthcare system were set up at the beginning of the 20th century. It gave more importance to an acute care approach and much less priority to prevention and public health. The main emphasis was on understanding and treating infectious diseases and reliance on laboratory research.[3]

This strategy made sense 100 years ago because of the prevalence of acute infectious diseases in a young population. However, it doesn't make any sense now. With the aging of the population, the burden of disease has shifted toward chronic diseases.

The most common causes of death are now obesity and smoking, which result in delayed but progressive disease.[4] Even in the developing world, chronic diseases are gradually outstripping acute infectious diseases.[5]

---

1 Fuster V, Kelly BB, editors. Promoting Cardiovascular Health in the Developing World: a critical challenge to achieve global health. Washington, D.C.: The National Academies Press, Institute of Medicine; 2010. https://www.ncbi.nlm.nih.gov/books/NBK45693/

2 https://www.ons.gov.uk/peoplepopulationandcommunity/birthsdeathsandmarriages/deaths/bulletins/deathsregistrationsummarytables/2018

3 Fleming D, William H. Welch and the rise of modern medicine. Boston, Massachusetts: Little, Brown; 1954.

4 Mokdad AH, Marks JS, Stroup DF, Gerberding JL. Actual causes of death in the United States, 2000. JAMA. 2004;291:1238–45. https://www.ncbi.nlm.nih.gov/pubmed/15010446

5 https://www.ncbi.nlm.nih.gov/books/NBK45693/

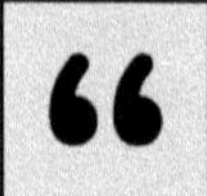

Really impressed with the service at AVID Clinic. I'm only part way through my treatment programme with them and my back pain has already greatly improved. Amazing customer service, everyone is very nice and welcoming. Would definitely recommend!

Becky Street

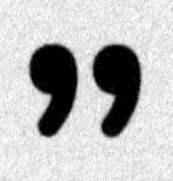

The main feature of modern healthcare is its use of a disjointed, task-based system that is aimed at addressing acute conditions. It takes notice only after asymptomatic persons become diseased and require drug treatment. This system favours speciality over primary care and procedures over cognitive tasks, for example, surgery instead of behaviour-change counselling.

Moreover, the modern healthcare system relies on new and costly technology even if its benefits are not clearly understood. Many preventive and cost-effective strategies are not researched or adopted because they cannot be patented or made profitable.

For example, between 2014 and 2020, total health spending in the UK has grown at 2% a year on average, from £124bn to £137bn. This period has seen constraints in NHS pay growth, staffing shortages, a marked rise in waiting times and rise in NHS provider deficits because the cost of delivering healthcare has outstripped funding. As a result, funding has focused increasingly on day-to-day spending at the expense of wider investment in the NHS.[6]

Modern medical research usually pursues isolated problems and short-term "magic bullet" solutions. Often, the model for treating acute infectious disease is applied to the treatment of chronic disease. For example, cancer chemotherapy is modelled after antibiotic therapy and coronary revascularization is modelled after abscess incision and debridement.

6 https://www.health.org.uk/news-and-comment/blogs/health-and-social-care-funding

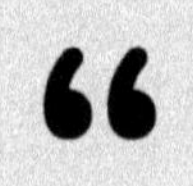

The process has been good so far, a really friendly team who are very warm and welcoming they have helped repair my lower back which was feeling horrible before and are putting my shoulders back in place I would recommend to anyone who has any back pain and is serious about there health and well-being.

Kamal John

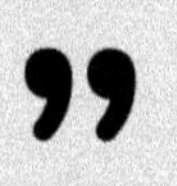

Changing this broken healthcare system requires alterations in medical education, medical research, health policy, and reimbursement. The current fragmentation of healthcare should be replaced by a patient-centred, whole-person approach. For example, the government should support research on the development and dissemination of prevention strategies. Moreover, it should reward the use of appropriate non-patentable therapies. Primary care physicians should act as health coaches and all healthcare professionals should adopt a coordinated multidisciplinary team approach.

Medical education should include prevention strategies such as lifestyle modification. Rather than only diagnosis and management of diseases, it should emphasize homeostasis, health, and the practice of cost-effective health promotion.

Although the need for management of acute disorders will remain, positive health promotion is the only way to halt the emerging pandemic of chronic disease.[7]

---

7 https://www.ncbi.nlm.nih.gov/pmc/articles/PMC4339086/

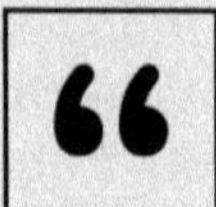

I have been seeing Trishul and their team at AVID Clinic for around a month now and honestly I could not fault the impeccable service, the outstanding treatment received and the absolutely fantastic advice I get with every visit to the Clinic. I have noticed thruout my treatment that my problems have improved completely, making me feel like a new man, being able to do things I couldn't have done before!

If I could give more than 5 stars I would! Thank you so much all at AVID Clinic for your warm smiles, laughs and always making me feel like family not just a client. I look forward to the next time I step in to the gorgeous Clinic!

Samuel Griffin

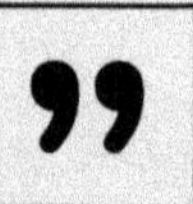

THE SICKCARE CRISIS

If our goal is to destroy the world—to produce global warming and toxicity and endocrine disruption—we're doing great.
~William McDonough

"I want to talk to you about one of the biggest myths in medicine, and that is the idea that all we need are more medical breakthroughs and then all of our problems will be solved."
~Quyen Nguyen

Our current healthcare system is focused not on health maintenance but on the treatment of disease, which is mainly dependent on expensive drugs and invasive surgeries. The mission of the present healthcare system seems to be to maximize profits rather than helping people to maintain or regain their health.[8]

8 http://articles.mercola.com/sites/articles/archive/2014/03/15/bad-american-health-care-system.aspx

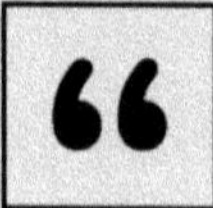

I first visited AVID Clinic some weeks ago and already have noticed a significant improvement with my back pain, movement and balance. I am looking forward to the end result in future weeks so I can play with my Grandchildren pain free!
Thank you AVID Team

Sharon Kirkness

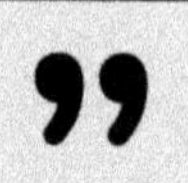

Not only is our health system mediocre-to-poor, but many of us are unable to access it easily. According to a large survey conducted by the Commonwealth Fund, the quality of healthcare attitudes and experiences of people across seven countries are ranked as follows:

1. Australia
2. Canada
3. Germany
4. New Zealand
5. the Netherlands
6. the United Kingdom
7. the United States

Hospitals also missed a series of key targets, including waiting times for cancer care and non-urgent operations, such as cataract removals, hernia repairs, and hip and knee replacements also took too long.

The highlights of the survey are:

1. **Fewer people are receiving healthcare**
   This is due to the high cost of modern medical care.
2. **Lack of regular, timed access to a primary healthcare provider**
   Often, doctors don't know important information about the medical history of their patients, which affects the quality of medical care.

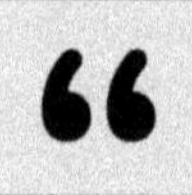

After the first week of having treatment I already feel better! The whole team are incredibly professional, friendly and helpful! The Clinic is a calm and welcoming environment and would highly recommend AVID to anyone who is need of an osteopath/chiropractor 10/10!

J Dawg

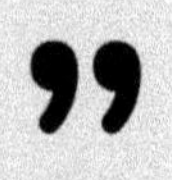

3. **Poor access to healthcare**
   For example, only 41 per cent of patients in the UK can consult a doctor on the same day that they need one. Access to after-hours medical care (early in the morning, late in the evening, and on weekends and holidays) is even more difficult. And one in six patients attending hospital A&E units had to wait longer than four hours.[9]

4. **Poor management of healthcare**
   This includes gaps in communication, duplicate testing, poor access to medical records, and violation of confidentiality.

5. **Medical errors**
   These include hospital-acquired infections, adverse drug reactions, inappropriate medical treatments, unnecessary surgeries, and operating on the wrong body part.

6. **Doctors don't listen to their patients**
   Patient satisfaction is also linked to how well their physicians explain things to them, how much time they spend with them and how well their appointments are managed.

7. **High chronic disease rates**
   This indicates a lack of attention to lifestyle habits such as diet, exercise, sleep, and stress management.

---

9 https://www.england.nhs.uk/statistics/statistical-work-areas/ae-waiting-times-and-activity/ae-attendances-and-emergency-admissions-2019-20/

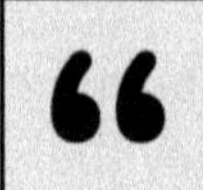

Would definitely recommend the AVID Clinic. I have suffered with shoulder and neck pain on and off for several years and after an initial consultation I started my treatments I'm already feeling the benefits. The staff are extremely professional and friendly, overall the Clinic has a lovely friendly vibe.

Lyn Isted

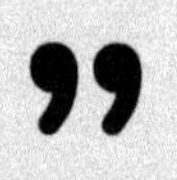

8. **Most people are dissatisfied with the current healthcare system**
   More than 15 per cent of Britons want a complete overhaul of the healthcare system. And only 26 per cent in the UK are satisfied with the present healthcare system.[10]

Some of the major problems of our healthcare system are:

1. CHRONIC DISEASE

One of the biggest health problems in the UK is **obesity**. The numbers are alarming.

- **64%** of UK adults are overweight or obese in 2017.
- Overall, **67% of men and 62% of women** are classified as overweight or obese.
- **20%** of children in Year 6 are classified as obese.
- **711,000** hospital admissions, where obesity was reported as a factor, up 15% from 2016/17.
- **10,660** hospital admissions directly related to obesity in 2017/18, only 100 less than in 2016.
- **29%** of adults are obese, up from 26% in 2016.[11]

10 Cathy Schoen, Robin Osborn, Michelle M. Doty, Meghan Bishop, Jordon Peugh and Nandita Murukutla. Toward Higher-Performance Health Systems: Adults' Health Care Experiences In Seven Countries, 2007. Commonwealth Fund in New York City

11 https://www.finder.com/uk/health-statistics

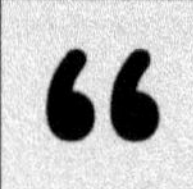

After months and months of suffering with severe lower back pain shooting down to my leg I decided to visit AVID. The AVID team have been so helpful to get me back walking normally again and I couldn't be more grateful for all the work they've put in! I would highly recommend AVID to anyone suffering from lower back pain.

Shyam Patel

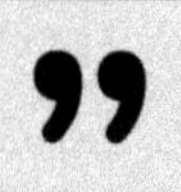

Unfortunately, the obesity epidemic has led to a more dangerous disorder: **metabolic syndrome**. The World Health Organisation and other medical groups, especially ATP-III, published the metabolic syndrome concept in 2002 to diagnose and treat an increased cardiometabolic risk. (It was formerly called **Syndrome X**.)

Metabolic syndrome consists of these five variables:

- obesity
- hyperglycemia (high blood sugar)
- hypertension (high blood pressure)
- hypertriglyceridemia and (high fat levels in the blood)
- low HDL[12] (low levels of good cholesterol)

According to the National Cholesterol Education Program High Blood Cholesterol ATP III guidelines, a person has metabolic syndrome if any three of the following are present:

Risk Factor	Defining Level
Abdominal obesity*	(waist circumference)
Men	>102 cm (>40 inches)
Women	>88 cm (>35 inches)
Fasting glucose	>110 mg/dL
Blood pressure	>130/>85 mmHg
Triglycerides	>150 mg/dL
HDL cholesterol	(mg/dL)
Men	<40 mg/dL
Women	<50 mg/dL

12 https://www.ncbi.nlm.nih.gov/pubmed/17469345

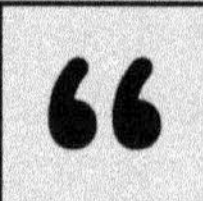

I went to the AVID Clinic with bad back problems and leg pains within 3 sessions I haven't had any leg pains and minimal back pain. I have continued my sessions the difference is amazing. the team are amazing with a fountain of knowledge behind them. Thanks very much guys

Barry Linsell

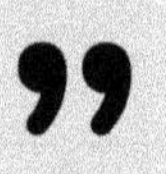

Risk factors for metabolic syndrome (minimum three)

**Overweight and obesity are associated with insulin resistance and metabolic syndrome. However, the presence of abdominal obesity is more highly correlated with metabolic risk factors than is an elevated body mass index (BMI). Therefore, the simple measure of waist circumference is recommended to identify the bodyweight component of metabolic syndrome.*

Metabolic syndrome is increasingly common, and up to one thirds of UK adults have it. The presence of metabolic syndrome or any of its components indicates a greater risk of developing complications such as type 2 diabetes and heart disease. However, positive lifestyle changes can delay or even reverse the development of serious health problems.

Another serious healthcare problem in the UK is **cancer**. Cancer is the leading cause of death in the UK, above heart disease and dementia.[13] Every day, nearly 990 people are diagnosed with cancer, and around 450 people die from the disease.[14] The number of new cancer diagnoses in England increased from 303,135 in 2016 to 305,683 in 2017 (excluding diagnoses for non-melanoma skin cancers).[15]

13 Public Health England (PHE). Health Profile for England: Chapter 2: major causes of death and how they have changed. London: PHE; 2018. Data from England & Wales, 2016

14 Calculated by the Cancer Intelligence Team at Cancer Research UK: based on all cancers combined excluding non-malignant melanoma (ICD10 C00-C97 exc. C44) in the UK in 2016.

15 https://www.ons.gov.uk/peoplepopulationandcommunity/healthandsocialcare/conditionsanddiseases/bulletins/cancerregistrationstatisticsengland/2017

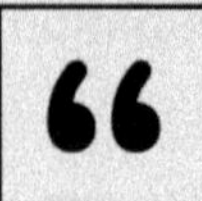

After having significant back issues consistently each year triggered by innocuous movements I was referred by a very good friend to see Trishul. I have been blown away by the feeling of being part of a wider family of practitioners and fellow sufferers and am now part way through treatment.

I look forward, always, to my visits and am already seeing a marked improvement in my movements and general pain as well as relief on tension headaches.

I couldn't recommend Trishul and his team more.

Michael Siggins

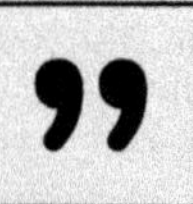

Furthermore, one in two people born after 1960 in the UK will be diagnosed with some sort of cancer during their lifetime.[16] And, by 2020, almost one in two people will get cancer at some point in their lives.[17] This rising incidence of cancer is an indication of a sick society in an unhealthy environment.

2. THE OPIOID CRISIS

Opioids are a group of pain-relieving drugs naturally found in the opium poppy plant. They can be made from the poppy plant (morphine) or synthesized in a laboratory (fentanyl). Opioids are suitable for relieving acute pain and pain at the end of life but there is little evidence that they are helpful for long-term pain.[18]

In fact, doctors that specialise in pain have stated that there is a lack of evidence of effectiveness and the potential for harm when opioids are prescribed for long-term pain.[19]

In spite of this, opioids are widely prescribed for long-term pain. Unfortunately, opioid prescribing more than doubled in the period from 1998 to 2018.[20]

---

16 Ahmad AS, Ormiston-Smith N, Sasieni PD. Trends in the lifetime risk of developing cancer in Great Britain: comparison of risk for those born from 1930 to 1960. British Journal of Cancer. 2015;112(5):943-947. doi:10.1038/bjc.2014.606. https://www.ncbi.nlm.nih.gov/pmc/articles/PMC4453943/

17 Macmillan Cancer Support (2013). Cancer mortality trends: 1992–2020. Estimated based on prevalence, incidence and mortality trends.

18 https://www.rcoa.ac.uk/faculty-of-pain-medicine/opioids-aware

19 https://www.bmj.com/content/352/bmj.i20

20 https://www.thelancet.com/journals/lanpsy/article/PIIS2215-0366(18)30471-1/fulltext

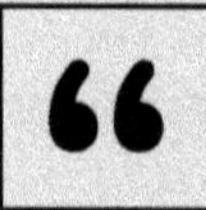

Trishul and the team are so friendly and I started to see results after the first few sessions! I highly recommend AVID Clinic!

Aiclia S

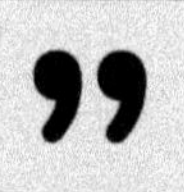

There is a reasonable fear of an opioid epidemic in the UK,[21] similar to the more serious opioid crisis in the USA.[22]

This clearly shows that our healthcare system is focusing on the symptom instead of the problem. Pain is just a symptom that tells us something is wrong. Pain is not the problem. Instead, we need to fix the real problem.

3. MENTAL HEALTH DISORDERS

Major depression is thought to be the second leading cause of disability worldwide and a major contributor to suicide and ischemic heart disease. Mental health in the UK is as follows:

- **1 in 6** people experienced a common mental health problem within the last week.
- **1 in 5 women** are reported to have mental health problems.
- **1 in 8 men** are reported to have mental health problems.
- **5,821** suicides were reported in the UK in 2017.
- **75%** of these suicides in the UK were by men.[23]

In addition, dementia and Alzheimer disease were the top cause of death in the UK in 2017 (12.7% of all deaths).

---

21 https://www.thetimes.co.uk/article/britains-opioid-epidemic-kills-five-every-day-83md7wc3k
22 https://www.hhs.gov/surgeongeneral/priorities/opioids-and-addiction/index.html
23 https://www.finder.com/uk/health-statistics

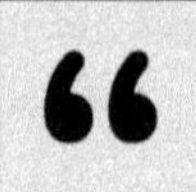

Highly recommend the AVID Clinic - after years of lower back pain I decided to get this sorted and came to the Clinic. After my initial consultation I came back for my first alignment and have never felt better.

I look forward to my weekly adjustments as the family friendly environment and the kind staff make is pleasure to visit the Clinic.

Now I'm road to recovery my only regret is that I didn't come sooner!

Kieran Bowling

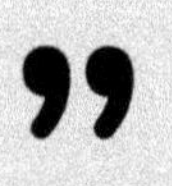

4. DECLINE IN QUALITY OF LIFE

Life expectancy of British adults has been cut by six months by the Institute and Faculty of Actuaries, which calculates life expectancy on behalf of the UK pension industry. The institute said it now expects men aged 65 to die at 86.9 years (instead of 87.4 years), while women who reach 65 are likely to die at 89.2 years (instead of 89.7 years). This is the biggest reduction in official longevity forecasts. Compared with 2015, projections for life expectancy are now down by 13 months for men and 14 months for women. Some of the possible reasons are austerity and cuts in NHS spending, and worsening obesity, diabetes and dementia.[24]

Stress: According to a survey on a study group of 2000 people across Great Britain, 37% of British residents feel stressed for at least one full day per week. Women were substantially more likely to be stressed than men; they suffered from stress for three more days per month than men. The most common cause of stress was money, followed by work, health concerns, failure to get enough sleep, and the pressure of household chores.[25]

Another UK-wide stress survey was commissioned by the ***Mental Health Foundation*** between 29th March and 20th April 2018. A total of 4619 adults were surveyed online. The results are representative of all UK adults (aged 18+). The study is believed to be the largest and most comprehensive stress survey in the UK.

---

24 https://www.actuaries.org.uk/news-and-insights/media-centre/media-releases-and-statements/longer-term-influences-driving-lower-life-expectancy-projections

25 https://www.forthwithlife.co.uk/blog/great-britain-and-stress/

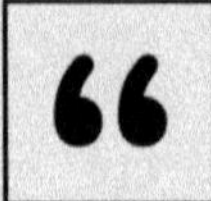

I can't rate AVID Clinic highly enough. Having visited here since August 2020 with sever pain in my back, I have been through an intensive programme for the last three months. Trishul is highly skilled and gives you regular updates during the treatment. I am now out of pain and can go about my daily life so much easier. The AVID Clinic is friendly, professional and a real asset to our community. You won't be disappointed. Give it a try.

Bev McGarey

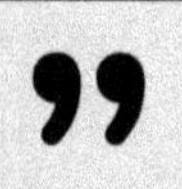

The highlights of the report:

- **74%** of UK adults felt so stressed at some point over the last year that they felt overwhelmed or unable to cope.
- **32%** of adults said they had experienced suicidal feelings as a result of stress.
- **16%** of adults said they had self-harmed as a result of stress.

The study is included in a new report by the Mental Health Foundation.

After the survey, Mental Health Foundation Director, Isabella Goldie said:

> *"Millions of us around the UK are experiencing high levels of stress and it is damaging our health. Stress is one of the great public health challenges of our time, but it still isn't being taken as seriously as physical health concerns.*
>
> *"Stress is a significant factor in mental health problems including anxiety and depression. It is also linked to physical health problems like heart disease, problems with our immune system, insomnia and digestive problems. Individually we need to understand what is causing us personal stress and learn what steps we can take to reduce it for ourselves and those around us.*[26]

Burnout: The World Health Organisation has now officially recognised burnout as an occupational phenomenon, describing it as a "syndrome resulting from chronic workplace stress that has not been successfully managed". It is characterized by

26 https://www.mentalhealth.org.uk/publications/stress-are-we-coping

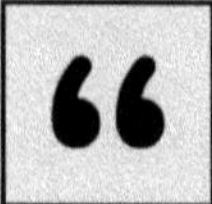

I came to AVID Clinic with neck and back pains. Surprised to see good result even after 1st treatment.

Further improvement achieved since then. Looking forward to full recovery with their help.

Harry Hanawa

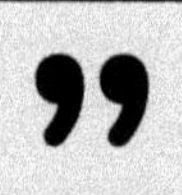

- feelings of exhaustion
- negativism or cynicism related to one's job
- poor work performance

Causes of burnout include unreasonable pressure, unmanageable workload, lack of support from managers, and toxic work culture.

Although statistics on the prevalence of burnout specifically are not available, 595,000 people in the UK suffered from workplace stress in 2018.[27]

27 https://www.bbc.com/worklife/article/20190610-how-to-tell-if-youve-got-pre-burnout

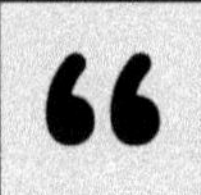

Incredibly friendly and welcoming but very professional too, a mix that is all too often missing these days. Highly recommended.

Stuart Scott

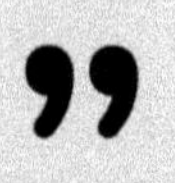

03

HEALTHCARE VERSUS SICKCARE

"We are not tinkers who merely patch and mend what is broken... we must be watchmen, guardians of the life and the health of our generation, so that stronger and more able generations may come after."
~Dr Elizabeth Blackwell (1821–1910), Anglo-American physician and the first woman doctor of medicine in modern times

"The enjoyment of the highest attainable standard of health is one of the fundamental rights of every human being without distinction of race, religion, political belief, economic or social condition."
~World Health Organization

Who is responsible for the state of our healthcare system? As Walter Cronkite wryly remarked, "America's healthcare system is neither healthy, caring, nor a system." That is why conventional healthcare is now called sickcare.

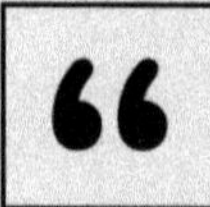

Came to AVID Clinic with lower back pain which I have had for over 20 years. I had a consultation and then later that day came back for a adjustment. The pain I have had for all those years went straight away. Was amazing standing up for the first time in years with no pain.

I've since been coming back and each time my back feels more inline and gain more movement.

My only regret is I never came sooner.

Lee Gregory

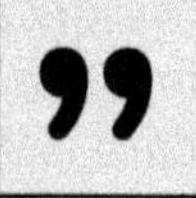

We tend to blame the following:

- **The government**, for mismanagement of the NHS, including budget cuts and the drive to privatise.[28]
- **The pharmaceutical industry**, for their exploitative and cynical marketing practices to GPs and members of the NHS.
- **The food industry**, for the production and promotion of highly processed, unhealthy foods.
- **The sick care system**, for its emphasis on crisis management instead of promotion of positive health practices

The goal of the sick care system is to take a patient from **–7 (strife) to 0 (survive)**. Its ideal is the "pain-free" state.

For example, if you have a disorder that affects your health, the sick care system will prescribe a drug that will relieve or reduce your symptoms. However, that drug probably won't eliminate the underlying cause of your disorder. So you may have to continue to take the drug as long as the disorder persists and you'll also have to deal with any side effects caused by it. And though you may have a slightly improved quality of life, you will have to depend on the drug to get through each day.

On the other hand, the goal of authentic healthcare is to transform every patient from **0 (survive) to +7 (thrive)**. Its ideal is "thriving", which means maximising performance and optimizing potential.

28 https://blogs.lse.ac.uk/politicsandpolicy/nhs-spending-on-the-independent-sector/

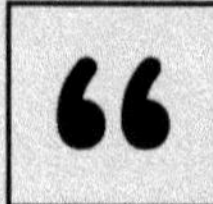

Great service by the team. Felt at ease from the start and provided a through treatment plan for my back and neck problems.

Peter Guntrip

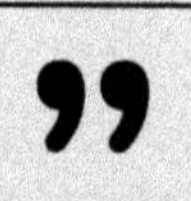

This ideal is in line with the World Health Organization's definition of health:

"Health is a state of complete physical, mental and social well-being and not merely the absence of disease or infirmity."[29]

The way I define health is the body's natural ability to heal.

This ideal of health can be best served by personalised medicine because it offers a combination of conventional medical therapies and complementary therapies that are backed by high-quality scientific evidence for safety and effectiveness. Personalized medicine is healing-oriented medicine that takes account of the whole person, including all aspects of lifestyle. It emphasizes the therapeutic relationship between practitioner and patient, is informed by evidence, and makes use of all appropriate therapies.[30]

I believe in personalised healthcare so that you can achieve the highest levels of your health. When you seek care with any of our team of healthcare experts at AVID Clinic, our goals during the initial stage are:

- Uncover the underlying cause of the health problem
- Suggest a care plan to produce the fastest results possible

---

29 Preamble to the Constitution of WHO as adopted by the International Health Conference, New York, 19 June - 22 July 1946; signed on 22 July 1946 by the representatives of 61 States (Official Records of WHO, no. 2, p. 100) and entered into force on 7 April 1948. The definition has not been amended since 1948.

30 The University of Arizona Center of Integrative Medicine. What is Integrative Medicine? https://integrativemedicine.arizona.edu/about/definition.html

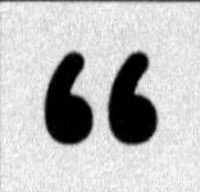

I attended my first appointment in pain and fed up due to not being able to run. Now feeling almost pain free and ready to lace up my running shoes again. Professional and friendly, every member of the team makes you feel welcome. I am more than happy with my treatment and the advice given is always valuable from exercises, new pillows to drink more hot chocolate - thanks everyone!

Rae Fogden

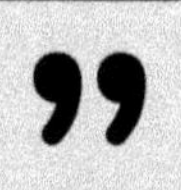

- Offer ways clients can participate in their recovery
- Explain the value of post-symptomatic wellness care

We help you to change the prevailing sickness care model of health (waiting for symptoms and then taking action) in favour of a bespoke wellness model that suits you. In this book, we will explain the vital principles that will help you to achieve your health goals. These are:

H – Hälsa

E – Exercise

A – Attitude Shift

L – Living Food

T – Time

H – Hydrate

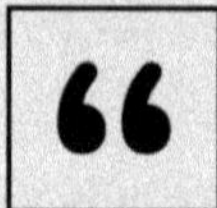

I started visiting AVID Clinic a few months ago after suffering with severe back problems for the last 20+yrs and having tried physio, acupuncture and various herbal remedies nothing worked until I started visiting Trishul. Starting a treatment plan with AVID was one of the best things I have done. I began to notice small changes to my mobility within the first couple of weeks. The staff couldn't be more helpful, I will definitely be continuing my treatment with them and would highly recommend AVID. Trishul is the Harvey Specter of his profession!

Misba Mirza

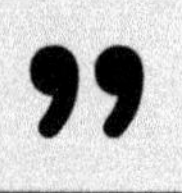

04

LIVE AVIDLY

"If there is a single definition of healing, it is to touch with mercy and awareness those pains from which we have withdrawn in judgment and dismay."
~Stephen Levine

"The preservation of health is easier than the cure of disease."
~Bartlett Joshua Palmer

AVID means "having or showing a keen interest in or enthusiasm for something", and it's the name of our company, **AVID Clinic**.

OSTEOPATHY

"An osteopath is only a human engineer, who should understand all the laws governing his engine and thereby master disease"
~Dr A.T. Still

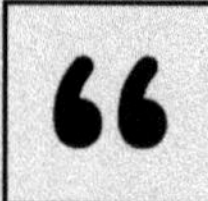

Been coming to AVID Clinic for the last couple of months, and I can honestly say i feel my aches and pains have gone and overall feeling a lot healthier and a lot more energetic.

All the staff are very accommodating and i would recommend to everyone.

Paul Johnson

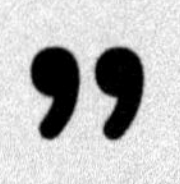

Osteopaths are trained in therapeutic approaches that are suitable for a broad range of individuals, including pregnant women, children and babies. Osteopathic care is delivered through a range of interventions which may include onward referral, health management advice, manual therapy, exercise therapy and others. Osteopaths adapt their therapeutic approach depending on the individual needs of the patient and their presenting complaint. Manual therapy techniques employed may include articulation and manipulation of joints and soft tissues.

Osteopaths have been regulated by statute since 1993 by the General Osteopathic Council (GOsC).

- Arthritic pain
- Circulatory problems
- Cramp
- Digestion problems
- Fibromyalgia
- Frozen shoulder/ shoulder and elbow pain/ tennis elbow (lateral epicondylitis) arising from associated musculoskeletal conditions of the back and neck, but not isolated occurrences
- Headache arising from the neck (cervicogenic)
- Joint pains
- Joint pains including hip and knee pain from osteoarthritis as an adjunct to core OA treatments and exercise
- General, acute & chronic backache, back pain (not arising from injury or accident)
- Generalised aches and pains
- Lumbago

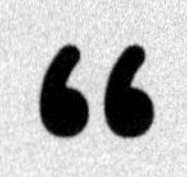

Brilliant and helpful. Very fun atmosphere and chilled experience. A huge relief on my shoulder, neck and lower back pain. Thank you for the support. Highly recommended.

Vik Kainth

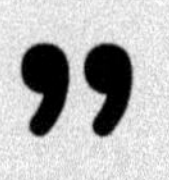

- Migraine prevention
- Minor sports injuries
- Muscle spasms
- Neuralgia
- Tension and inability to relax
- Rheumatic pain
- Sciatica
- Uncomplicated mechanical neck pain (as opposed to neck pain following injury i.e. whiplash)

CHIROPRACTIC

"I've been going to chiropractors for as long as I can remember.
It's as important to my training as practicing my swing."
~Tiger Woods

"Look well to the spine for the cause of disease"
~Hippocrates

Chiropractic comes from Greek and means "done by hand." The practice originated in the late 1890s with Daniel David Palmer, a self-taught healer in Iowa. He sought a cure for illness and disease that did not rely on drugs or surgery. Palmer reported curing deafness in a man who had lost his hearing after straining doing heavy work. Palmer attributed the hearing loss to a displaced vertebra and treated it by adjusting the man's spine.

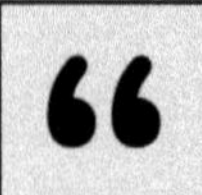

Knowledgeable staff who are friendly and invested in your health and well-being. Keep up the amazing work!

Rob Lawrence

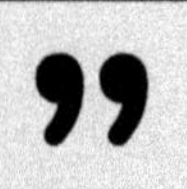

Based on this and other cases he treated with spinal adjustments, Palmer advanced his theory that most disease is caused by misaligned vertebrae that impinge on spinal nerves. Such misalignments are called subluxations. According to Palmer, correcting these misalignments reestablishes normal nerve and brain function and allows the body to heal itself.

Through advancements in research and a deeper understanding of how the body works, the "bone out of place causing disease" theory has been debunked. However, what we have learnt is that when the spine is not moving correctly (the causes of which can be physical, chemical or emotional), the brain then receives a distorted image of what the body is doing and how it is functioning. This then results in a state of miscommunication, misinterpretation and maladaptation, placing the body into a state of "stress" and dysfunction. It has been shown that through specific, targeted and repeated adjustments of the spine, the brain and body become better "connected" resulting in an optimized state of function and maximized potential. This has been shown to vastly improve the quality of life and reduce the symptoms so many patients present with.

Many chiropractors focus on musculoskeletal problems of the spine, that is, conditions affecting the backbone and associated muscles. Chiropractors most commonly adjust the spine by using their hands to apply forceful pressure on areas that are out of alignment or that do not have normal range of motion. Chiropractors also use mobilization (manual therapy that does not involve a high-velocity thrust) as well as physical therapy.

Although spinal manipulation is the key component of chiropractic care, practitioners take a holistic approach and include such things as nutrition counselling and exercise advice in their treatment program.

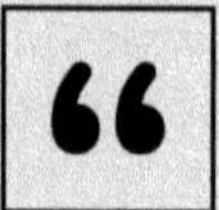

Amazing experience, very welcoming and done an amazing job to know everything about me and how he would help relieve the pain 10/10

Jack Saunders

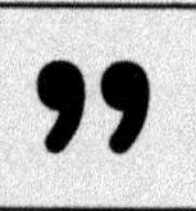

Chiropractic care is the most commonly used form of complementary and alternative medicine. Chiropractors are the third largest group of healthcare providers, after physicians and dentists, who treat patients directly. The American Medical Association (AMA) policy now states that it is ethical for physicians not only to associate professionally with chiropractors but also to refer patients to them for diagnostic or therapeutic services.

Family practitioners were the most likely physicians to refer to chiropractors, followed by family nurse practitioners, internists, neurologists, neurosurgeons, gynaecologists, and general surgeons. Chiropractors also frequently refer patients to other healthcare providers.[31]

Chiropractors are able to treat and manage:

- Ankle sprain (short term management)
- Cramps
- Elbow pain and tennis elbow (lateral epicondylitis) arising from associated musculoskeletal conditions of the back and neck, but not isolated occurrences
- Headache arising from the neck (cervicogenic)
- Joint pains
- Joint pains including hip and knee pain from osteoarthritis as an adjunct to core OA treatments and exercise
- General, acute and chronic backache, back pain (not arising from injury or accident)

31 Christensen MG, Kollasch MW, Hyland JK. Practice analysis of chiropractic, 2010. A project report, survey analysis, and summary of the practice of chiropractic within the United States. Greeley, CO: National Board of Chiropractic Examiners; 2010

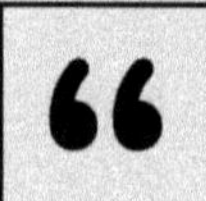

This Clinic is beautiful, with everything under one roof. Dr Trishul Vadi is very professional and his team were excellent. Received a full consultation and treatment same day. 5 stars!

Felicity Bugess-Young

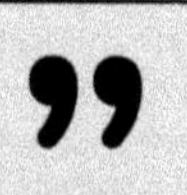

- Generalised aches and pains
- Lumbago
- Mechanical neck pain (as opposed to neck pain following injury i.e. whiplash)
- Migraine prevention
- Minor sports injuries
- Muscle spasms
- Plantar fasciitis (short term management)
- Rotator cuff injuries, disease or disorders
- Sciatica
- Shoulder complaints (dysfunction, disorders and pain)
- Soft tissue disorders of the shoulder
- Tension and inability to relax

Regulated by the General Chiropractic Council (GCC) in the UK, the profession is growing rapidly, with more and more seeking out chiropractic care to reduce pain and maximise the potential in their lives.

PHYSIOTHERAPY

Physiotherapy is a well-established profession and takes a whole-person approach to health and well-being, which includes our general lifestyle. Physiotherapists use movement and exercise, manual therapy, education and advice to help people affected by injury, illness or disability. They help to manage pain, restore movement and function and prevent disease.

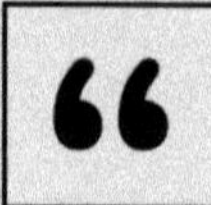

I've been coming to AVID forever and always leave better than when I stepped through the door.

Andrew MacFarlane

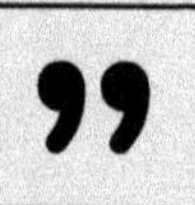

You can benefit from physiotherapy at any time in your life. Physiotherapy enables people to stay in work while helping them to remain independent for as long as possible. More importantly, it encourages you to be an active participant in your own treatment.

Physiotherapy is a degree-based healthcare profession. Physiotherapists use their knowledge and skills to improve a range of conditions associated with different systems of the body, such as:

- Neurological disorders like stroke, multiple sclerosis, and Parkinson's disease
- Neuromusculoskeletal disorders like back pain, whiplash associated disorders, sports injuries and arthritis
- Cardiovascular disorders like chronic heart disease, and rehabilitation after a heart attack
- Respiratory disorders like asthma, chronic obstructive pulmonary disease, and cystic fibrosis.
- Post-operative rehabilitation

Physiotherapists work in a variety of health departments and social care. They are involved in education, research and service management.[32]

Top Benefits of Physiotherapy

Physiotherapists can help you to:

- manage pain
- avoid surgery
- prevent injuries
- recover from a stroke

---

32 https://www.csp.org.uk/careers-jobs/what-physiotherapy

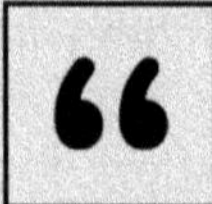

Great place. Staff very friendly and helpful. Overall a great place to come & get the help for neck and back pain.

Claudia Chadwick

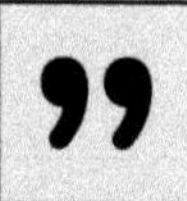

- maximize your movement
- improve mobility and balance
- improve performance in sports
- manage heart and lung disease
- manage age-related health conditions
- regain original physical abilities and skills
- avoid or reverse dependence on pain medication
- manage diabetes and its complications like peripheral neuropathy[33]

At AVID Clinic we believe in a multi-care evidence based approach, where the whole team works together and are directly or indirectly involved in your care to address the needs of your body. This multi-care view is our "secret sauce" of how we are able to give amazing results over and over again.

VITALISM

Vitalism means to believe in the body's innate ability to heal itself. It recognises and respects the intelligent order in the universe and body (in comparison to a state of unorganised chaos). It recognises that through order and harmony, life is fully expressed. Vitalism acknowledges that if there is interference of this order, a state of dis-ease will be the result.

33 https://www.movementforlife.com/blog/top-5-key-benefits-of-physical-therapy.php

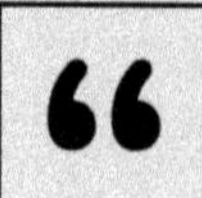

An excellent service. Trishul has maintained my health levels and is always available for any other advice. I would highly recommend AVID Clinic and my friends Trishul and Komal.

Kevin Browne

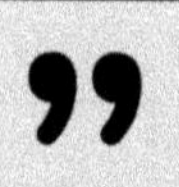

According to Life University, "Our bodies work hard to express health, to maintain health, and to recover from illnesses or other conditions that threaten our health." For Chiropractors in a vitalistic paradigm of thought, the primary objective of an adjustment is to allow restoration of order, by allowing the intelligent brain to view the body correctly and thus allow healing to occur the natural way that it should.

It is easier to believe in vitalism when you are young. Your body is youthful and resilient. In this state of mind, you do not doubt your body's ability to return to health, you simply let it get on with it, without interference.

As an alternative philosophical view, mechanism sees the body as a set of mechanical systems such as the pulmonary or cardiovascular systems and treats those systems as separate entities. Mechanism is best understood as a reference to allopathic medicine. Where symptoms are addressed as a primary focus, and once symptoms are reduced and managed, intervention or continued treatment is stopped.

There are elements of truth in both vitalism and mechanism. You can honour the body's ability to participate in its own healing. At the same time, you can respect what mechanists do and look for ways to work with those ideas instead of against them. Let common sense and the facts guide you to a rational decision. Give importance to evidence-informed and patient-centred medicine. Focus on what works and is supported by Clinical evidence. Indeed, the best treatment should be based on the best available evidence and the best results.[34]

34 https://www.chiroeco.com/vitalism-vs-mechanism-a-fresh-view/

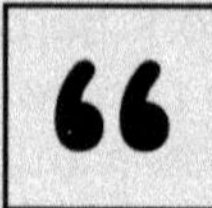

Great personal service from Trishul and the team. When I met them I was very restricted in my movement with aches and pains everywhere!

Couple of months of treatment and now I am well on the road to recovery

Many thanks to all the team

Highly recommend

Steve Franco

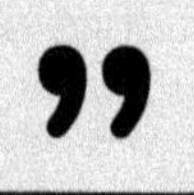

At AVID Clinic, we have a vitalistic view towards health. We respect and understand the role of a mechanistic viewpoint, and work with all colleagues in healthcare. Our goal is simply to bring our patient to health.

HEALTH IN THE COMMUNITY

"The power of community to create health is far greater than any physician, Clinic or hospital."
~Dr Mark Hyman

"The need for connection and community is primal, as fundamental as the need for air, water, and food."
~Dr Dean Ornish

A healthy community is one in which groups from all parts of the community work together to prevent disease and establish healthy living options. Community-level healthcare brings the greatest health benefits to the greatest number of people. It also helps to reduce health gaps caused by differences in income, education, race and ethnicity, location and other factors.

To improve the health of your community, start by taking care of your own health and the health of your family. Ensure that you are as healthy as possible with the help of healthy nutrition, daily physical activity, and regular check-ups.

Then help to promote health in your community by becoming more engaged in your community. Encourage local community groups and government organizations to consider community health in their plans.[35]

35 https://blogs.cdc.gov/publichealthmatters/2015/09/a-healthy-community-is-a-prepared-community/

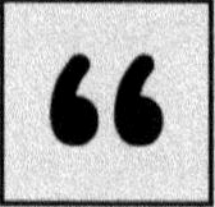

Great place, really friendly. I've been coming for 6 weeks to help with my Migraines which I've had for 30+ years. Since coming, No Migraines 😀. Should have done this years ago.

Stuart Pope

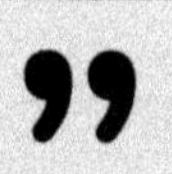

Promoting and maintaining a healthy community is everybody's business and the responsibility of every individual living in it. In the words of Coretta Scott King, "The greatness of a community is most accurately measured by the compassionate actions of its members."

HEALTH IN THE FAMILY

"Medicine cannot function without family."
~Carol Levine

The importance of family for wellbeing

The importance of family is evident in healthcare. Family support can provide comfort, support, and even influence better health outcomes while you are not well. Families establish patterns of preventive care, exercise, hygiene, and responsibility. They also set the foundation for self-worth, resilience, and the ability to form healthy and caring relationships.[36]

The healthiest, longest-living people in the world all have something in common: they put their families first. One of the biggest challenges for families to stay connected is the busy pace of life. Author Mimi Doe recommends connecting with your family by spending time together and expressing love and support to one another. Also, it's important to let go of little grievances.[37]

The same practices apply to close friends as well. This is especially important if you don't have a living family or stay far away from your family.

36 https://www.takingcharge.csh.umn.edu/create-healthy-lifestyle/relationships/why-relationships-family-are-important/-importance-family-wel

37 https://www.takingcharge.csh.umn.edu/nurture-your-relationships

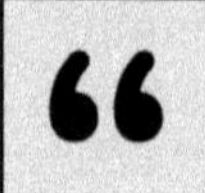

Great place, very friendly staff!

So pleased to not need to click my neck anymore. My back and neck are so much better since I started coming to AVID Clinic.

Katie Hind

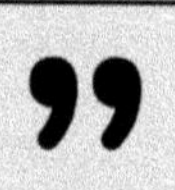

LOVE AND HEALTH

"The best and most beautiful things in this world cannot be seen or even heard, but must be felt with the heart."
~Helen Keller

"Far too many people are looking for the right person, instead of trying to be the right person."
~Gloria Steinem

According to a growing body of scientific research, love gives you exceptional health benefits. Dr Helen Riess, director of the Empathy and Relational Science Program at Massachusetts General Hospital, lists these five health benefits of love:

1. **Love makes you happy.**
   When you first fall in love, dopamine, the feel-good brain chemical associated with reward, is activated. It makes you feel positive and appreciated and this naturally is good for your health.
2. **Love busts stress.**
   After the initial phase, another brain chemical, oxytocin or the bonding hormone is activated. It reduces stress levels and creates greater homeostasis and balance.
3. **Love eases anxiety.**
   Being in love and feeling close to another person can reduce the anxiety about loneliness and insecurity.
4. **Love makes you take better care of yourself.**
   Couples encourage each other to go to the doctor when they don't want to. Sometimes, partners will even notice early signs of health problems before the sufferer.

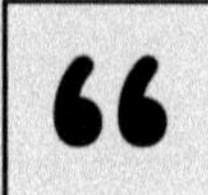

Such a wonderful team, right from the warm welcome at the start, through to Trishul and his professionalism. Wholeheartedly recommended to those suffering with spinal issues.

Anish Dholakia

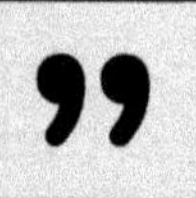

5. **Love helps you live longer.**
   Research has shown that married couples enjoy greater longevity than singles because of consistent social and emotional support and better adherence to medical care.[38] Also, a partner can hold you accountable to a healthy lifestyle and steer you away from unhealthy behaviour. Married couples have lower rates of substance abuse,[39] and lower blood pressure and less depression[40] than singles.[41]

In the words of Sophocles, "One word frees us of all the weight and pain of life. That word is love."

38 https://time.com/3706692/do-married-people-really-live-longer/
39 https://www.ncbi.nlm.nih.gov/pmc/articles/PMC1449833/
40 https://academic.oup.com/abm/article/35/2/239/4569261
41 https://time.com/5136409/health-benefits-love/

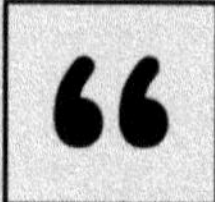

Amazing friendly environment, caring staff. After coming for 6 months the improvement in my back and hips is immense, walking the dog is a pleasure...

Sarah Mulhern

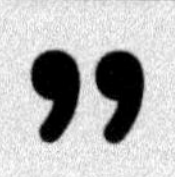

05

EXERCISE-THE ENERGIZER OF LIFE

"The body will become better at whatever you do, or don't do. You don't move?
The body will make you better at NOT moving.
If you move, your body will allow more movement."
~Ido Portal

"To wild animals, movement is not a chore, not a temporary punishment for being physically lazy and out of shape, not an optional activity just for better looks."
~Erwan Le Corre

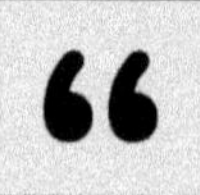

I came with a bad shoulder, it was getting more and more uncomfortable day by day. After my first few appointments I could noice the difference. Pain was decreasing and my back straighter. This was priceless. If you have a problem, just come in and see the staff, they are so friendly and have your best interest at heart.

Matthew Gundry-White

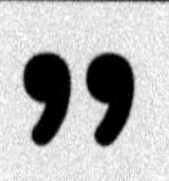

MODERN MAN MOVEMENT VERSUS PRE-INDUSTRIAL MAN MOVEMENT

Before the Industrial Revolution, strenuous physical activity was a normal part of the daily lives of our ancestors. They worked hard to gather food and to provide shelter and safety to the community. But their physical exertion was not limited to the requirements of their work life. In those days, people engaged in 1- or 2-day periods of intense and strenuous exertion, followed by 1- or 2-day periods of rest and celebration.

However, even during these so-called rest days, they made 6- to 20-mile round-trip visits to other villages to see relatives and friends and to trade with other clans or communities. They also took part in dancing and other social activities.[42]

Today, our physical activity is much lower than our pre-industrial age ancestors. Thanks to modern technology, we have low levels of physical activity and high levels of sedentary behaviour. According to WHO estimates, about one in five adults were not active enough in 2010 globally (20% of men and 27% of women).[43]

“In less than two generations, physical activity has dropped by 20% in the UK and 32% in the U.S. In China, the drop is 45% in less than one generation. Vehicles, machines and technology now do our moving for us.

42 U.S. Department of Health and Human Services. *Physical Activity and Health: A Report of the Surgeon General*. Atlanta, GA: U.S. Department of Health and Human Services, Centers for Disease Control and Prevention, National Center for Chronic Disease Prevention and Health Promotion, 1996

43 https://www.who.int/news-room/fact-sheets/detail/physical-activity

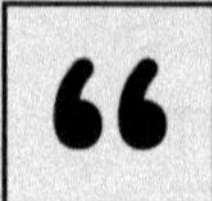

I came to see Trishul at his Clinic with back and neck problems. I had to ice my back every day otherwise I would get sciatica and my shoulders were incredibly tight to the poi t where I was forever tipping my head to one side or another, trying to stretch the muscles.

After just a couple of visits my neck issues had subsided significantly. Furthermore, after around three quarters of my scheduled visits my back had improved to the point where I did not need to ice it every day. In fact I managed two holidays without needing to put anything on my back.

I just want to say a big thank you to Trishul and his Clinic for working some magic on my wonky bits!

John "Johnnie" Hamilton

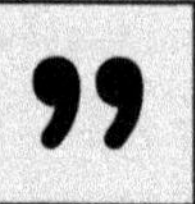

What we do in our leisure time doesn't come close to making up for what we've lost."[44]

The biggest challenge that prevents us from walking or doing other kinds of physical activity is lack of time. Regular aerobic physical activity has to compete with the demands of home, work, school and community.

WE ARE DESIGNED TO MOVE AND NOT TO BE STILL

"The truth about the human species is that in body, spirit, and conduct we are designed to grow and develop in ways that emphasise rather than minimize childlike traits. We are intended to remain in many ways childlike; we were never intended to grow "up" into the kind of adults most of us have become."
~Ashley Montagu

The human body works best when it's active. From an evolutionary perspective, we were designed to move—to move about and engage in all manner of manual labour throughout the day. This was essential to our survival as a species. The recent shift from a physically demanding life to a sedentary one has been relatively sudden.

Moreover, during the past 20 years, the time we spend in front of screens (smartphones, computers, television and video games) and driving personal vehicles has increased dramatically. The health consequences of a sedentary life cannot be reversed by exercise. Therefore, we have to reduce our total sitting time in addition to regular moderate-to-intense exercise.

44 https://www.icsspe.org/bookshop/designed-move

I am currently going through the treatment at AVID Clinic and could not recommend them enough. Great place with lots of lovely people. Super professional & great at their job!

Gintare Jankunaite

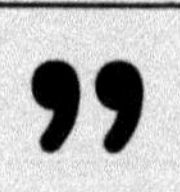

Parents often tell their children to go out and play. Adults need similar advice from their physicians![45]

SITTING VERSUS STANDING

"Sitting is the new smoking."
~Dr. James Levine

Sitting too long has also been linked to a higher risk of earlier death.[46] Sitting for extended periods leads to contracture of the abdominal and hamstring muscles and affects the lower back. Using a standing desk for a while can help to maintain better spinal alignment and muscle symmetry. However, standing all day is also not ideal. Taking frequent breaks is the best way to ensure you're standing or sitting optimally. Also, take care of your posture: the top of the computer screen should be about eye level.

Breaking up sitting with standing or short walks relieves pain and fatigue and improves control of blood sugar, blood pressure and weight gain. Watching television or playing games while standing is also a good way to reduce sitting time. However, the potential advantages of standing as opposed to sitting need to be further studied.[47]

TYPES OF EXERCISE AND THEIR BENEFITS

"If you only have time to exercise or meditate but not both, then make exercise your daily meditation."
~Steve Pavlina

45 https://www.ncbi.nlm.nih.gov/pmc/articles/PMC2996155/
46 http://annals.org/aim/article-abstract/2653704/patterns-sedentary-behavior-mortality-u-s-middle-aged-older-adults
47 https://www.healthline.com/health-news/debate-over-standing

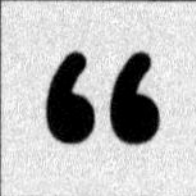

I only wish I had come here sooner - in a very short space of time I felt free of pain and continue to improve. Very friendly and professional staff who always so welcoming. They even surprised me with cake and a card on my birthday.

Wendy Fitzgerald

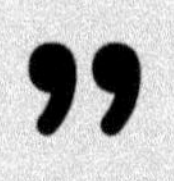

Strengthening, stretching, balance, and aerobic exercises are the four most important types of exercise, which will keep you active, mobile, and feeling great.

1. Aerobic exercise

Aerobic exercise speeds up your heart rate and breathing and increases endurance. Aim for 150 minutes per week of moderate-intensity activity such as brisk walking, swimming, jogging, cycling, dancing, or classes like step aerobics.

2. Strength training

As we age, we lose muscle mass. Strength training builds it back. Strengthening your muscles not only makes you stronger, but also stimulates bone growth, lowers blood sugar, helps weight control, improves balance and posture, and reduces stress and pain in the lower back and joints. Strength training includes bodyweight exercises like squats, push-ups, and lunges, and exercises against resistance from a weight, a band, or a weight machine.

3. Stretching

Ageing leads to a loss of flexibility in the muscles and tendons. Stretching helps to improve flexibility, increases your range of motion, and reduces pain and the risk for injury. You need to stretch all parts of your body every day. Warm up your muscles first, and then perform static stretches for up to 60 seconds of the calves, thighs, lower back, shoulders, arms, and neck.

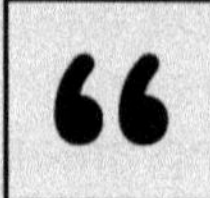

I love the team at AVID Clinic, they have been exceptional during my treatment.

Trishul was the first osteopath/chiropractor who gave me a realistic timeframe in which I would have my back fixed, and he was right! I couldn't recommend highly enough

Liam Hinds

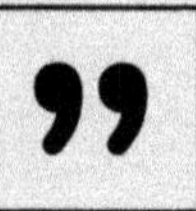

4. Balance exercises

Improving your balance helps prevent falls, which is especially important as we get older. If you have a fear of falling, consult a physical therapist, who will determine your current balance abilities and prescribe specific exercises to target your areas of weakness. Balance exercises include standing on one foot or walking heel to toe, with your eyes open or closed, and walking on uneven surfaces. Yoga or tai chi classes are also good options to improve balance.[48]

Most people tend to focus on one activity or type of exercise and think they're doing enough. However, each type of exercise is different. Doing them all will give you more benefits. Mixing it up also helps to reduce boredom and cut your risk of injury. Also, some activities fit into more than one category. For example, many endurance activities also build strength. And some strength exercises can also help improve balance and flexibility.[49]

1. YOGA

Yoga is a mind and body practice that combines physical postures, breathing exercises, and relaxation. Yoga develops flexibility, endurance, balance, and muscle strength. Practising yoga has been shown to increase mindfulness not just in class but also in other areas of a person's life. Yoga is now being included in many cardiac rehabilitation programs due to its cardiovascular and stress-relieving benefits.

48 https://www.health.harvard.edu/exercise-and-fitness/the-4-most-important-types-of-exercise
49 https://go4life.nia.nih.gov/4-types-of-exercise/

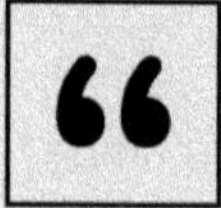

I've been attending the AVID Clinic for about 6 weeks now and it's has been a very positive experience. The whole team are professional and caring. I've noticed a significant improvement in my issues - highly recommend.

Hilary Nelson

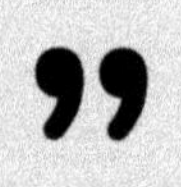

There are many types of yoga. Hatha yoga (a combination of many styles) is one of the most popular types. Hatha yoga focuses on *pranayamas* (breath-controlled exercises), *asanas* (yoga postures), and *savasana* (a resting period).[50]

2. PILATES

Pilates is named after its creator, Joseph Pilates, who developed the exercises in the 1920s. Pilates is a method of exercise that consists of low-impact flexibility and muscular strength and endurance movements. Pilates emphasizes proper postural alignment, core strength and muscle balance. Many Pilates exercises can be done on the floor with just a mat.

The health benefits of Pilates include:

- Improved core strength and stability
- Improved posture and balance
- Improved flexibility
- Prevention and treatment of back pain

However, Pilates doesn't include aerobic exercise so you will need to complement it with aerobic exercises such as brisk walking, running, biking or swimming.[51]

3. SWIMMING

Swimming is great exercise because you have to move your whole body against the resistance of the water. Swimming is a good all-round activity because it:

50 https://www.health.harvard.edu/staying-healthy/yoga-benefits-beyond-the-mat

51 https://www.mayoClinic.org/healthy-lifestyle/fitness/in-depth/pilates-for-beginners/art-20047673

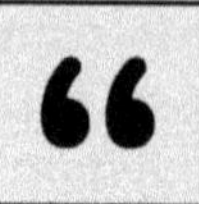

I've had osteopathic and facial aesthetic treatments at the Clinic over the last 5 weeks and can honestly say that both Komal and Trishul have been superb and the results of treatments have been beyond what I expected. With regards to the facial aesthetics treatment, everything was explained very clearly and carried in such a relaxed manner that there was very little , if any, discomfort at all . Friends and colleagues have asked 'have you been away ? ,You look very well, you look rested ' without realising I've had treatment, and that is exactly what I wanted ; for no one to actually figure out what I've done.

The ongoing osteopathic treatment has been such a success in a short space of time that I no longer worry climbing up or down stairs , and my posture has improved greatly.

Thank you to the whole team , including the wonderful reception staff , for making such a positive impact on my life.

Dr Pratish Dholakia

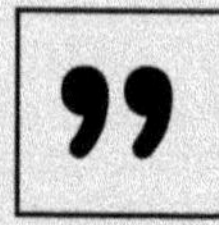

- builds endurance, muscle strength and cardio-vascular fitness
- tones muscles and builds strength
- helps maintain a healthy weight, healthy heart and lungs
- provides a full-body workout, as almost all your body muscles are used during swimming.[52]

However, the swimming pool can be used not only for swimming but also for water aerobic exercises such as water walking, running, or jogging and vigorous aerobic exercises. Heated pools can help to warm up your joints and muscles. And aquatic exercise can improve physical functioning in adults over 50.[53]

4. RUNNING

Studies have shown that running can help prevent obesity, type 2 diabetes, heart disease, high blood pressure, stroke, some cancers, and many other disorders. The health benefits of running include:

- It helps you live longer
- It helps you lose or maintain weight
- It improves the quality of your emotional and mental life
- It reduces your risk of cancer.[54]

52 https://www.betterhealth.vic.gov.au/health/healthyliving/swimming-health-benefits
53 https://www.mayoClinic.org/healthy-lifestyle/fitness/in-depth/ready-to-get-in-on-the-aquatic-fitness-movement/art-20390059
54 https://www.runnersworld.com/beginner/a20847956/6-ways-running-improves-your-health-0/

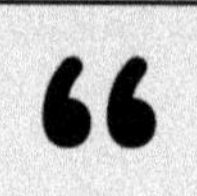

The Clinic has focussed on the injury I sustained in an accident and remarkable improvements have been experienced in shoulder pain and walking movement. Additional improvements experienced in heart health after six months of chiropractic treatment. Now working on developing strength. I explored some beauty therapy but I was not a suitable subject for that. I trust their assessments. All staff are warm and welcoming and the rooms are light and attractive. I continue to attend as I experience ongoing wellbeing.

Marion Small

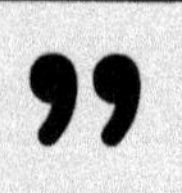

Even 5 to 10 minutes a day of low-intensity running is enough to extend life by several years, compared with not running at all.[55] And the sweet spot for maximum longevity is up to 2.5 hours of running a week.[56]

5. STRENGTH TRAINING

Strength training should be an important part of every fitness program. It helps you to reduce body fat, increase lean muscle mass and burn calories more efficiently. Strength training also helps you to:

- develop strong bones
- reduce or maintain your weight
- enhance your quality of life
- reduce the signs and symptoms of many chronic conditions, such as arthritis, back pain, obesity, heart disease, depression and diabetes.
- sharpen your thinking and learning skills and improve your memory.

Strength training can be done at home or in the gym using:

- bodyweight exercises such as push-ups, pull-ups, planks, lunges and squats.
- free weights such as barbells and dumbbells.
- resistance tubing, which is lightweight tubing that provides resistance when stretched.
- exercise machines[57]

55 http://content.onlinejacc.org/article.aspx?articleID=1891600
56 http://aje.oxfordjournals.org/content/early/2013/02/27/aje.kws301.full
57 https://www.mayoClinic.org/healthy-lifestyle/fitness/in-depth/strength-training/art-20046670

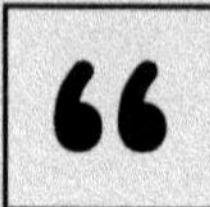

This is such a great Clinic to have found, Trishul and his team are extremely knowledgable and welcoming. And he is working wonders with my back! Would highly recommend

Andrew Boyle

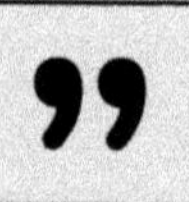

6. CROSSFIT

CrossFit is a training program that builds strength and conditioning through extremely varied and challenging workouts. In CrossFit, everyone has to do the same workout each day.

Most CrossFit gyms will split their classes into three or four sections:

- Dynamic warm-up. It consists of jumps, jumping jacks, jump rope, squats, push-ups, lunges, pull-ups, functional movements, stretches, and mobility work.
- Skill or Strength work. If it's a strength day, you'll work on a pure strength movement like squats or deadlifts. If it's not a strength day, you'll work on a skill like one-legged squats.
- Workout of the day. You will either do a certain number of reps of particular exercises as quickly as possible or have a set time limit to do as many of a certain exercise as possible.
- Cool down and stretch. You're allowed to stretch out on your own or as a group.

A word of caution: CrossFit is not for everyone. If you have a history of injuries or medical conditions, it may not be the best choice for you. Most CrossFit gyms will let you attend one class for free. If you have a few in your area, try out each of them once before choosing the one that suits you best.[58]

58 https://www.nerdfitness.com/blog/a-beginners-guide-to-crossfit/

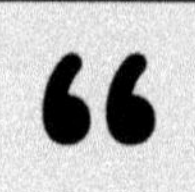

The level of care that I receive is excellent! Pain relief was gained within about two sessions and what's equally as important, I'm moving towards a stronger and healthier body. Thank you Trishul.

Margaret Pierre

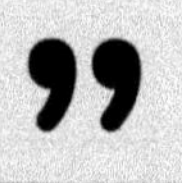

7. ZUMBA

Zumba is a fitness program that combines Latin and international music with dance moves. Zumba can be moderate or vigorous aerobic activity, depending on the intensity. It incorporates interval training (alternate fast and slow rhythms) and resistance training. The class gives you a powerful cardio workout and also builds your coordination and agility. Zumba dance moves are easy to follow and easy to learn. It's a full-body workout that is adaptable for any fitness level. The music, energetic environment, group experience and changing routines will have you sweating but in a fun way.[59]

8. CORE EXERCISES

You use your core muscles to do everyday activities like tying your shoes and lifting heavy objects. It also affects your balance, posture, and stability.

The core includes your abdominal muscles as well as the muscles in your back and around your pelvis. Strengthening these muscles helps to stabilize your body, support your spine, and enhance your overall fitness. If you have a past or current back injury, consult a personal trainer. They can show you how to safely tone and train your core.[60] Core exercises for beginners include the plank, crunches, bicycle crunch, leg raises, push-ups, and boat.[61]

59 https://www.mayoClinic.org/healthy-lifestyle/fitness/expert-answers/zumba/faq-20057883

60 https://www.healthline.com/health/best-core-exercises

61 https://www.stylecraze.com/articles/core-strengthening-exercises

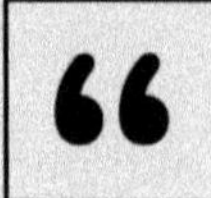

Went in for my adjustment, feel a completely new person. Wonderful service, felt very welcome and comfortable. Highly recommended!

Richard Djan-Krofa

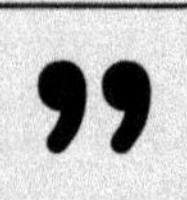

9. FINE MOTOR CONTROL

Fine motor control is the ability to make small, precise movements, such as picking up a tiny object with your thumb and index finger. Damage to the brain, nerves, muscles or joints due to injury, illness, and stroke can impair fine motor control. They can also be impaired by congenital deformities, cerebral palsy, or developmental disabilities.

Therapeutic exercises can help to improve damaged fine motor control functions. For example, the Stroke Association recommends the following exercises:

- **Forced Use:** Constraint-induced movement therapy is an effective exercise for the loss of fine motor control. For example, if you've lost the use of your right hand, you may revert to using your left hand. During constraint-induced movement therapy, your left hand is tied to your side, forcing you to rely on your impaired limb for all your fine motor actions. This exercise may be used for up to six hours a day.
- **Timing:** Choose a task such as inserting pegs in holes. Start a timer and fill all the holes. Repeat the exercise every day, aiming for faster times each day until you reach your optimum ability.[62]

WHEN SHOULD YOU EXERCISE?

The best time for exercise is different for each person. Work out at the time that is most suitable for you. The key is to do what's most likely to work for you because consistency is more important than timing.

62 https://www.sportsrec.com/126568-occupational-therapy-exercises-fine-motor.html

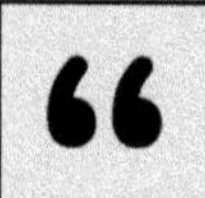

Highly recommend coming to see Trishul if your having back problems, only been coming for a month or so but feel so much better, staff are so friendly feel very welcomed

James Paul

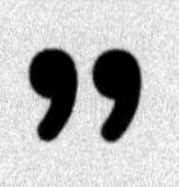

For example, you might have heard that the best time to exercise is early in the morning. But if you're not a morning person, you may find it difficult to get up early to work out. Similarly, if you find that working out late in the evening keeps you from falling asleep easily, you may have to exercise earlier in the day or try less intense forms of movement. Finally, if your schedule isn't predictable or you are travelling, you may need to be flexible and exercise whenever possible.

There's no one right time of day to exercise. So do it at the time that's best for you.[63]

DOES EXERCISE HAVE TO CHANGE WITH AGE?

We tend to underestimate and undermine the physical potential of elders. They can definitely exercise, even if they have diminished flexibility and functional capacity due to age and sedentary lifestyle. However, they should consult your doctor before starting any exercise regimen, including a review of pre-existing diseases and current medications.

Motivation: Many seniors are anxious, tense, and nervous in an exercise setting, which may make them reluctant to try something new or different. However, most of them understand the dangers of inactivity and the benefits of exercise. Their exercise program should be individualized so that they feel confident and secure. It is important to be supportive because elders often feel self-doubt and uncertainty.

63 https://www.heart.org/en/healthy-living/fitness/fitness-basics/when-is-the-best-time-of-day-to-work-out

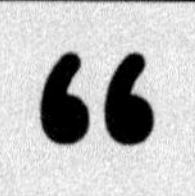

Regularly go for back adjustments which keep me mobile and motivated for my martial arts challenges but also now see Komal for all my dental treatment. She is meticulous, thoughtful, and caring, and I feel like I am in safe hands. Have had pain free fillings to the point I didn't even notice the injection.

I certainly feel like a member of the family at AVID Clinic.

Dom Boydell

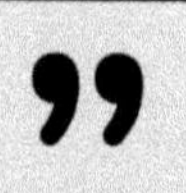

Safety: Safety is the most important concern with elder exercise programs. They should exercise in well-lighted areas with user-friendly equipment. It is important for them to drink water before, during and after exercise to avoid dehydration. They may also have to wear layered clothing to adjust to varying temperatures. They need to slow down and stop if they experience any health warning signs during exercise such as breathing difficulty or fatigue.

Set Realistic Goals: Before starting an exercise program, it is important to set individualized, realistic, and attainable goals. They should start with low to moderate level activity. The overall goal should be to improve strength, flexibility, body composition and cardiovascular endurance.

Warm-up and Flexibility: Each session should be started with a warm-up session such as walking and stretching all the joints for 10-15 minutes. Similarly, the session should be ended with a cool-down period, which includes stretching and relaxation.

Aerobic Exercise: Aerobic activities such as walking, swimming, aqua exercise and cycling are all suitable for elders. Swimming and aqua exercise cause less stress on the joints. Similarly, stationary cycling places less stress on the joints, while recumbent cycling puts less stress on the back. Walking at a higher pace than normal walking can be easily done in most environments and requires no additional equipment.

Strength Training: Muscular strength, functional mobility and balance can be significantly improved with resistance training under supervision. Elders can do a resistance exercise program three days per week. They should be reminded to breathe regularly and not to hold their breath during resistance exercises.

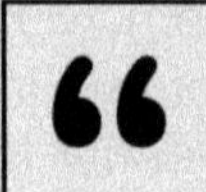

Had a great experience. The whole team are very welcoming. Wouldn't have any hesitation in recommending anyone to use Trishul and his team.

Dr Heera Farmah

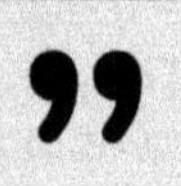

A sedentary lifestyle leads to disability, early death, and a low quality of life. Chronological age does not represent quality of health. A range of opportunities for lifetime fitness is available for seniors of all ages. Preventing the complications associated with inactivity is far more cost-effective than the costs of long-term care.[64]

BEST RECOMMENDATIONS

"If we had a pill that contained all of the benefits of exercise, it would be the most widely prescribed drug in the world."
~Dr. Ronald Davis

- Move more and sit less to offset the risk of heart disease, high blood pressure, and mortality due to increased sedentary behaviour. Set a timer and stretch or take a short walk every 30-45 minutes.
- Move more frequently throughout the day. Integrate more movement into your daily life. Take the stairs instead of the lift. Walk short distances. Exercise while watching TV. Walk while talking on your mobile phone.

Optimize your health

For the best health benefits from physical activity, you need at least 150 to 300 minutes of moderate-intensity aerobic activity like brisk walking or fast dancing each week. You also need to do muscle-strengthening exercises like push-ups or lifting weights, at least 2 days each week.[65]

64 https://www.unm.edu/~lkravitz/Article%20folder/age.html
65 https://health.gov/paguidelines/second-edition/10things/

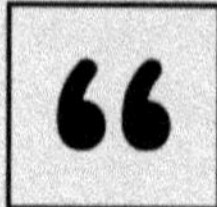

After suffering with pain in my back for about a year, I had resigned myself to the fact that it would just be something I had to live. Gradually the pain got worse which is when I went to see Trishul Vadi at the AVID Clinic. After a thorough examination, Trishul completely understood the problem and put in place a plan of action over the next 3 months. Within 2 weeks the pain had already started to subside. Trishul works wonders and I would highly recommend him and his very friendly team at the AVID Clinic.

Amy Hobbs

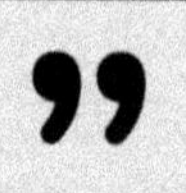

Aerobic exercise and strength training are both important for improving your endurance and muscle mass. You also need to improve your flexibility and balance. Finding the right balance will depend on your individual goals, how quickly you want to achieve them, and the amount of time you can commit to exercising.[66]

Final thought:

"If all people understood how to use water, one-half of all the afflictions from disease would be removed. The other half would be taken care of by understanding how and when to eat, how to breathe and the necessity of daily exercise."
~Louisa Lust

66 https://www.healthline.com/health/how-often-should-you-work-out

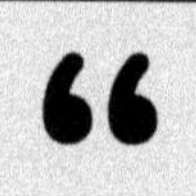

A fantastic Clinic with first class service.

Having received osteopathy treatment for the past two months for chronic lower back pain my condition has now greatly improved and my quality of life has also too!

The AVID Clinic team are very professional and I would not hesitate to recommend them to anyone who is thinking of receiving such treatment in the future.

Mark Loveland

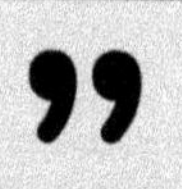

06

AVID-TUDE SHIFT- THE EMPOWERER OF LIFE

"The greatest revolution of our generation is the discovery that human beings, by changing the inner attitudes of their minds, can change the outer aspects of their lives."
~William James

"A healthy attitude is contagious but don't wait to catch it from others. Be a carrier."
~Tom Stoppard

MIND-BODY CONNECTION

"The brain and peripheral nervous system, the endocrine and immune systems, and indeed, all the organs of our body and all the emotional responses we have, share a common chemical language and are constantly communicating with one another."
~Dr James Gordon (founder of the Center for Mind-Body Medicine)

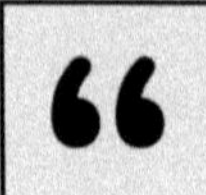

Very warm welcoming staff and atmosphere. Although only 3 weeks into treatment, marked improvements have been noticed. Sleep pattern has greatly improved too. Look forward to seeing the end result!

Joy Akah-Douglas

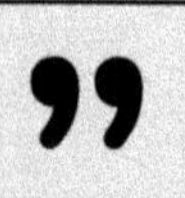

The mind-body connection means that our thoughts, feelings, beliefs, and attitudes can affect the functioning of our body positively or negatively. On the other hand, what we eat, how much we exercise, and even our posture can affect our mental state, positively or negatively. This results in a complex interplay between our minds and bodies.

Mind-body therapies use the body to influence the mind and vice versa. These include

- Meditation
- Prayer
- Yoga
- Tai chi
- Qigong
- Biofeedback
- Relaxation
- Hypnosis
- Guided imagery
- Patient support groups
- Cognitive behavioural therapy
- Creative arts therapies (art, music, or dance)

It's important to note that the mind is not the same as the brain.

- The mind consists of mental states such as thoughts, emotions, beliefs, attitudes, and images. (software)
- The brain is the organ that allows us to experience these mental states. (hardware)

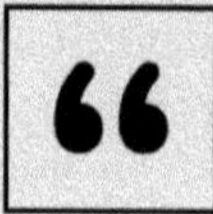

Has made a massive difference to my quality of life when the NHS could offer no help at all! I am more mobile and stronger than before. Thank you for getting me back to normal and keeping me there!
I can now be the active mum
I wanted to be for so long!

Amanda Wolf

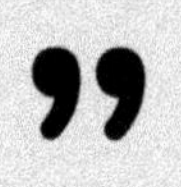

Mental states can be conscious or unconscious. Each mental state causes a positive or negative effect in the physical body. For example, the mental state of anxiety causes the production of stress hormones. Many mind-body therapies help you to become more conscious of your mental and emotional states. You can then use this awareness to guide your thoughts and emotions in a better and more positive direction.[67]

WHAT IS A HEALTHY MIND?

"The key to a healthy life is having a healthy mind."
~Richard Davidson

A healthy mind is not merely the absence of mental disease. According to the World Health Organization (WHO), mental health is "a state of well-being in which the individual realizes his or her own abilities, can cope with the normal stresses of life, can work productively and fruitfully, and is able to make a contribution to his or her community."[68]

Mental health is a dynamic state of internal stability that enables us to use our abilities in harmony with the universal values of society. The components of a healthy mind are

- a harmonious relationship between body and mind
- basic cognitive and social skills

---

67 https://www.takingcharge.csh.umn.edu/what-is-the-mind-body-connection

68 World Health Organization. Promoting mental health: concepts, emerging evidence, practice (Summary Report) Geneva: World Health Organization; 2004

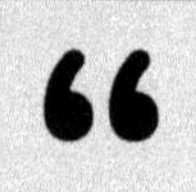

Fantastic friendly staff, that helped with getting my health back on track, would highly recommend to anyone who has even the slightest of back problems

Ben Webb

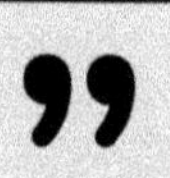

- the ability to recognize, express and control our own emotions
- the ability to empathize with the emotions of others
- the ability to fulfil different social roles and
- the ability and flexibility to cope with adverse life events[69]

Some steps you can take to develop a healthy mind:

- **Be active**
  Movement and exercise boost your mood. They also help you to sleep better and get the rest you need.
- **Lower your alcohol intake**
  Alcohol can increase feelings of depression and also affect your physical health.
- **Connect with family and friends**
  Quality time with your loved ones is the best way to boost your mental wellbeing.
- **Be open and curious**
  Learn a new sport, language, learn to play an instrument, read books and feed your mind with positive inspiration.[70]

Positive affirmations

Positive affirmations are positive phrases or statements used to reverse negative or unhelpful thoughts. They can be used to decrease stress, boost your self-esteem or to bring about positive changes in your life.

---

69 https://www.ncbi.nlm.nih.gov/pmc/articles/PMC4471980/
70 https://www.sahealth.sa.gov.au/wps/wcm/connect/Public+Content/SA+Health+Internet/Healthy+living/Healthy+mind/

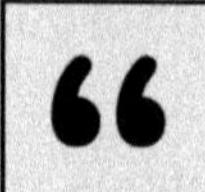

I can feel a remarkable difference in my back. I feel like a brand new woman and the pain has completely gone from my uppper back which has caused me havoc for years. I highly recommend Trishul.

Dipika Pattni

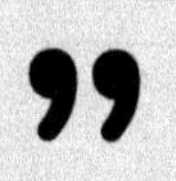

Practising positive affirmations is simple. Pick a positive phrase that resonates with you and repeat it to yourself. However, positive affirmations require regular practice if you want to make sustainable long-term changes.

Positive affirmations are designed to encourage an optimistic mindset. They reduce negative thoughts and the tendency to linger on negative experiences

When we replace negative messages with positive statements, we can construct more hopeful narratives about who we are and what we can accomplish.

Positive affirmations are based on the idea that your thoughts can influence your health for the better. They can be used to improve physical health as well as to heal emotional pain.

For example, these are a few of author Louise Hay's positive affirmations:

1. Life brings me only good experiences. I am open to new and wonderful changes;
2. I feel glorious, dynamic energy. I am active and alive;
3. Every experience I have is perfect for my growth;
4. Today I create a wonderful day and a wonderful new future;
5. Abundance flows freely through me;
6. My self-esteem is high because I honour who I am.[71]

---

71 https://www.louisehay.com/affirmations/

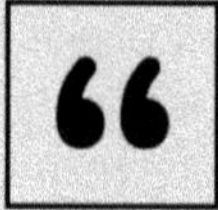

It's excellent because of the friendly service. Trishul takes the pain away.

Kevin Clarke

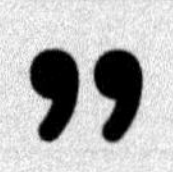

Whether you're seeking a means of dealing with stress or just want to improve your emotional state, use the above or create your own affirmations.[72]

PAIN—THE MENTAL COMPONENT

"Pain is inevitable; suffering is not." ~the Buddha

Pain is defined as "an unpleasant sensory and emotional experience associated with actual or potential tissue damage, or described in terms of such damage". Pain is a sensation of the body and is always an unpleasant emotional experience.

Pain is the leading reason for patients seeking medical care and is one of the most disabling, burdensome, and costly conditions. Pain accompanies many diseases, each one of which generates separate diagnostic, therapeutic and research problems.[73]

The following factors can affect our perception of and reaction to pain:

1. our existing beliefs about pain
2. our beliefs about our ability to control pain (self-efficacy)
3. earlier experiences of pain
4. expectations of recovery
5. current emotional states, including catastrophizing, anxiety, and depression)[74]

72 https://positivepsychology.com/daily-affirmations/
73 https://www.ncbi.nlm.nih.gov/pubmed/25000837
74 https://www.physio-pedia.com/Psychological_Basis_of_Pain

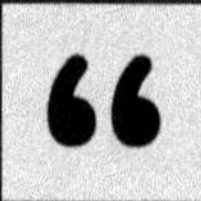

Highly recommend Trishul.

He made a a great job to treat my sciatica

Thanks a lot

Bertrand Fontenier

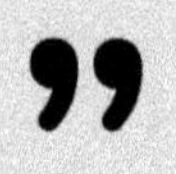

Mindful meditation involves focusing the mind to increase awareness of the present moment. This method to help cope with pain and stress can be easily done anywhere. An example of mindful meditation would be to sit up straight, close your eyes, and focus your attention on your incoming and outgoing breathing. This exercise could be done for just a couple of minutes or longer. It helps you to let your thoughts come and go while being aware of your respiration. It can be most helpful during stressful times and difficult life events.

Mindful meditation can create a sense of control, which helps you to make your experience of pain more manageable. Yoga, tai chi and other mind-body techniques are also recommended to get the same benefits.[75]

COGNITIVE BEHAVIOURAL THERAPY

Cognitive behavioural therapy (CBT) is a talking therapy that can help you manage your problems by changing the way you think and act. It's most commonly used to treat anxiety and depression. However, it can also be useful for other mental and physical health problems.

CBT is based on the concept that your thoughts, feelings, physical sensations and actions are interconnected. CBT aims to help you deal with overwhelming problems in a more positive way by breaking them down into smaller parts. You're shown how to change your negative patterns to improve the way you feel. CBT deals with your current problems, rather than focusing on issues from your past. It looks for practical ways to improve your state of mind every day.

75 https://www.hss.edu/conditions_emotional-impact-pain-experience.asp

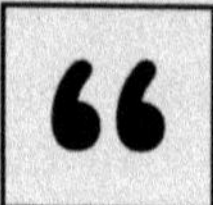

Amazing place, staff can't do enough to make you feel welcome. Most importantly though my course of chiropractic treatments is working, and I'm feeling better after each visit. Can't recommend highly enough.

Thomas Blaza

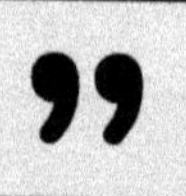

Uses of CBT

CBT is an effective way of treating a number of different mental health conditions. In addition to depression or anxiety disorders, CBT can also help people with:

- bipolar disorder
- borderline personality disorder
- eating disorders – such as anorexia and bulimia
- obsessive-compulsive disorder (OCD)
- panic disorder
- phobias
- post-traumatic stress disorder (PTSD)
- problems related to alcohol misuse
- psychosis
- schizophrenia
- sleep problems – such as insomnia

CBT is also sometimes used to treat people with long-term health conditions, such as irritable bowel syndrome (IBS), chronic fatigue syndrome (CFS) and fibromyalgia

Although CBT cannot cure the physical symptoms of these conditions, it can help people cope better with their symptoms.

Cognitive behavioural therapy (CBT) can be as effective as medicine in treating some mental health problems, but it may not be successful or suitable for everyone.

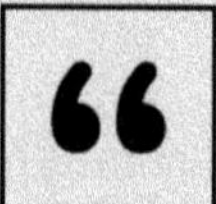

Great service, lovely people, clean and modern facilities, and actual improvement with my back pain ! Cannot recommend highly enough

Saint Anger

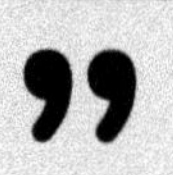

Benefits of CBT:

- it may be helpful in cases where medicine alone has not worked
- it can be completed in a relatively short period of time
- it can be provided in different formats, including in groups, self-help books and apps
- it teaches useful and practical strategies that can be used in everyday life, even after the treatment has finished

Drawbacks of CBT:

- You need to commit yourself to the process to get the most from it – a therapist can help and advise you, but they need your cooperation.
- It can take up a lot of your time.
- It may not be suitable for people with more complex mental health needs or learning difficulties.
- It involves confronting your emotions and anxieties so you may experience initial periods where you're anxious or emotionally uncomfortable.
- It focuses on the person's capacity to change their thoughts, feelings and behaviours. CBT does not address any external circumstance that may affect your health and wellbeing.[76]

76 https://www.nhs.uk/conditions/cognitive-behavioural-therapy-cbt/

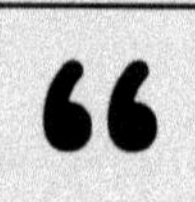

Great support, very friendly staff. Would recommend AVID Clinic to anyone

Kim Godbeer

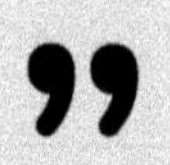

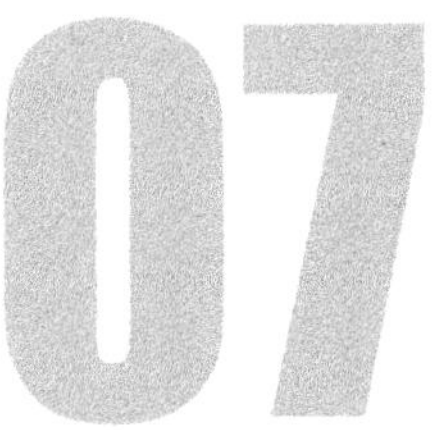

LIVING FOOD-THE ESSENCE OF LIFE

"A healthy outside starts from the inside."
~Robert Urich

"The food you eat can be either the safest and most powerful form of medicine or the slowest form of poison."
~Ann Wigmore

YOU BECOME WHAT YOU EAT

"You are what you eat, so don't be fast, cheap, easy or fake."
~Unknown

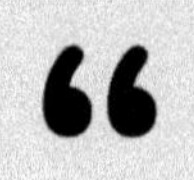

Great care and service from Trishul and his team.

Gina Hajitheodosi

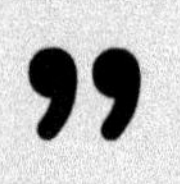

The proverbial saying 'You are what you eat' means that you need to eat good food to be fit and healthy. It's literally true because the structure and function of every cell in your body depend on the nutrients in your food. You are constantly repairing and rebuilding your body. Every cell in your body has a fixed lifespan. Your body is busy making new cells to replace those that have died. The health of these new cells depends on the quality of your diet. A nutritious and healthy diet can help you build healthy cells.[77]

FAD DIETS AND THEIR DOWNFALL

"Any food that requires enhancing by the use of chemical substances should in no way be considered a food."
~John H. Tobe

Fad diets may offer an easy way to reduce weight but they are usually unsuitable, unsustainable or unsafe. It is advisable to consult your doctor before attempting any such diet.

Some of the worst fad diets in history are

- the clay diet
- the air diet
- the tapeworm diet
- the cookie diet
- the Fletcherizing diet
- the sleeping beauty diet
- the cotton ball diet[78]

---

77 https://cynthiasass.com/sass-yourself/sass-yourself-blog/item/116-why-you-really-are-what-you-eat.html
78 https://www.freshnlean.com/7-worst-fad-diets-history/

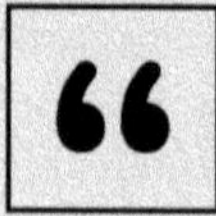

I went to see Trishul at AVID Clinic to get some advice about my neck and back and general posture and received some amazing feedback. I was given a warm welcome and really liked how comfortable I was made to feel from the start.

Trishul did a examination which was quick, and gave me a really detailed and understandable explanation of my problems and outlined the structure of the treatment which was really clear and took into consideration many other restrictions I had, financial / time wise.

If you want a professional, relaxed and friendly environment with unambiguous explanations of treatment - get yourself to AVID Clinic!

Joshan Mahmud

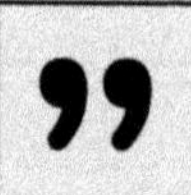

Features of fad diets

- They have rigid and irrational rules. For example, eating predominantly one type of food such as grapefruit, meat or cabbage soup.
- They require the elimination of entire food groups such as carbs or fats.
- They promise rapid weight loss of two pounds a week or more.
- They severely restrict calories
- They are frequently promoted by celebrities.

Jumping from one fad diet to another may result in yo-yo dieting. Making small sustainable changes that will last a lifetime is much more effective and healthy.[79]

MEAT VERSUS VEGETARIAN VERSUS VEGAN

"Pay the farmer or pay the hospital."
~Birke Baehr

Most people in the UK eat meat, but this number appears to be decreasing. Though vegetarians and vegans make up around 3% of the population, 24% of people in a recent survey described their dietary status as 'other' than non-vegetarian, vegan and lacto-ovo-vegetarian. Flexitarian diets (flexibly vegetarian or semi-vegetarian), are becoming more popular.

79 https://mayoClinichealthsystem.org/hometown-health/speaking-of-health/dont-fall-for-a-fad-diet

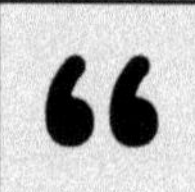

Highly recommend Trishul for his chiropractic care. He provides a detailed diagnosis and recommended treatment plan. Staff at the Clinic are very welcoming and helpful. 5 stars to everyone at AVID Clinic keep it up.

Jean Azzopardi

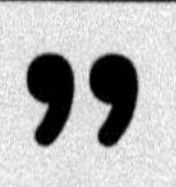

People become vegetarians for many reasons, including health, concerns about religious convictions, the use of antibiotics and hormones in livestock, concerns about animal welfare, or to avoid excessive use of environmental resources. Some people can't afford to eat meat. Also, becoming a vegetarian has become easier because of the availability of more vegetarian dining options, fresh produce, and the influence of Asian cultures with largely plant-based diets.

Meat is a good source of protein, B vitamins and minerals such as iron, selenium and zinc. However, meat is high in saturated fat. Also, the consumption of red and processed meat is linked with an increased risk of bowel cancer. In the UK, the recommendation is to eat less than 500 g/week of cooked meat and to choose lean meats.

Vegetarian and vegan diets consist mainly of fruit, vegetables, whole grains, beans, pulses, lentils, nuts, and seeds. They contain very little saturated fat and are rich in dietary fibre. This may be why vegetarian and vegan diets are associated with lower risks of obesity, high blood pressure, type 2 diabetes, heart disease and cancer. According to the American Dietetic Association, "Appropriately planned vegetarian diets, including total vegetarian or vegan diets, are healthful, nutritionally adequate, and may provide health benefits in the prevention and treatment of certain diseases."

It is not clear whether these health benefits are due to one particular element of the diet or of all the parts together. Or if it is because vegetarians and vegans are more health conscious and make healthier lifestyle choices such as being more active and avoiding smoking and excess alcohol consumption. However, eating more fruits and vegetables is likely to have significant health benefits.

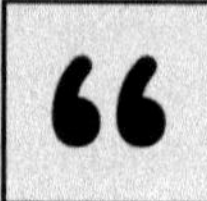

I have used AVID Clinic for the last 4 year. I was having great difficulty walking and came to AVID Clinic. That has been the best decision I've made. I was able to get around and am very active as a result. I have continued with maintenance treatment now.

Marlene Dermer

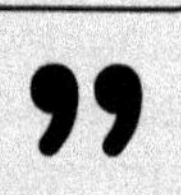

Balanced vegan or vegetarian diets can be a healthy choice. People decide to go meat-free for many different reasons. However, it may not be necessary to cut out meat completely for health reasons. A plant-based diet includes all diets that emphasise fruits, vegetables, plant-based proteins and whole grains. For example, the Mediterranean diet comprises plenty of fruits and vegetables, beans, nuts, cereals, unsaturated fats (such as olive oil) but also fish and smaller amounts of dairy and meat products.

Plant-based eating is promoted in many national healthy eating guidelines, including the UK's own *Eatwell Guide*.[80] Shifting our current diet to the eating pattern presented in this guide would result in an estimated 32% lowered carbon footprint, thus improving our health as well as helping the environment.[81]

RAW VERSUS PROCESSED

"Came from a plant, eat it; was made in a plant, don't."
~Michael Pollan

We are the only animals that process our food. Processed foods are foods that are no longer in their natural state because they have been cooked or combined with other food ingredients. For example, raw peanuts are in their natural state. However, roasted peanuts are no longer in their natural state because they have been cooked.[82]

80 https://www.nhs.uk/Livewell/Goodfood/Pages/the-eatwell-guide.aspx
81 https://www.nutrition.org.uk/bnf-blogs/meatfree.html
82 http://www.bioedonline.org/lessons-and-more/lessons-by-topic/ecology/resources-and-the-environment/raw-vs-processed-food/

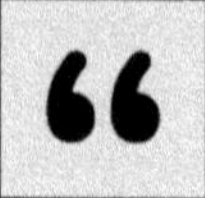

I couldn't recommend AVID Clinic more!! Its not just the calming environment or the wide range of treatments they offer, but the staff are just fantastic! I couldn't fault AVID if I tried. I went to see Trishul for chiropractic treatment for a back injury and he had me up and moving after the first appointment. Each appointment from then on had me feeling better and better. He was beyond helpful and also a very funny guy which made me feel really relaxed. I also got to meet his lovely wife Komal, who was so kind and helpful when I first arrived for my emergency appointment.
Thank you all so much!

Dr Vidhi Patel

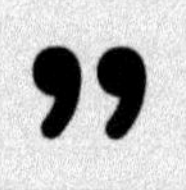

A raw-food diet consists of mostly raw plant foods such as raw fruits and vegetables, nuts, seeds, fermented foods and sprouted grains. It is made up of at least 70% raw foods, which are mostly unheated, uncooked and unprocessed.

Benefits of a raw food diet:

- Cooking foods deactivates the enzymes in them. However, there is no evidence that food enzymes contribute to better health.
- Some nutrients, particularly water-soluble vitamins, are lost during the cooking process.
- Raw fruits and vegetables may contain more nutrients like vitamin C and B vitamins.

Drawbacks of a raw food diet:

- Cooked foods are easier to chew and digest than raw foods.
- Cooking your vegetables may make some antioxidants more available to your body than they are in raw foods.
- Cooking food effectively kills bacteria that may cause food-borne illnesses. This applies especially to meat, eggs and dairy.

Neither a completely raw nor completely cooked diet can be justified by science. That's because both raw and cooked fruits and vegetables have various health benefits, including a lower risk of chronic disease.[83]

Some foods are more nutritious when eaten raw, while others are more nutritious after being cooked.

---

83 http://cebp.aacrjournals.org/content/13/9/1422

Following a car crash I had serious pain in my neck, back, shoulder and elbow. I have never been to an osteopath, chiropractor or anything like this before so I didn't know what to expect or whether it would work for me. I came to Trishul at AVID Clinic and in the first session he located where the pain was coming from and explained really clearly with a lot of knowledge about what was going on in my back to cause the pain, he could also tell me things about my body without me even telling him. He is always friendly and willing to impart knowledge with me and is very clear in his explanations. My treatment has been amazing, I'm no longer in pain, I am training harder and better, recovering quicker and thinking clearer. This really has been the best thing I've done for myself and if I could give AVID 10 stars I definitely would

Nancy Tsang

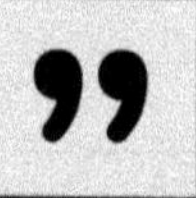

- Foods that are healthier raw: broccoli, cabbage, garlic, onions
- Foods that are healthier cooked: asparagus, carrots, legumes, mushrooms, potatoes, spinach, tomatoes, meat, and fish and poultry

Eat a combination of cooked and raw foods for maximum health benefits. However, it's unnecessary to follow a completely raw diet for good health.[84]

MAKE BETTER FOOD CHOICES

"Let food be thy medicine, and thy medicine thy food."
~Hippocrates

Make your health a priority and take time to care for yourself.

1. Get personalized nutrition information based on your age, gender, height, weight, and physical activity level.
2. Enjoy your food but eat less. Use a smaller plate at meals to help control the amount of food and calories you eat. Eat slowly and mindfully.
3. Make half your plate fruits and vegetables. Choose red, orange, and green vegetables like tomatoes, sweet potatoes, and broccoli, along with other vegetables. Eat fruit for dessert.
4. Drink water throughout the day to help maintain a healthy weight. Avoid soft drinks and alcohol.
5. Choose whole grains like brown rice and whole-grain pasta and bread more often. Foods with high-fibre content provide key nutrients and also give you a feeling of fullness.

84 https://www.healthline.com/nutrition/raw-food-vs-cooked-food

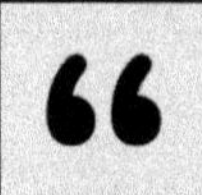

The entire team at AVID Clinic are brilliant, I have been a customer for many years and come for a variety of treatments and services. I have recommended AVID to friends and family who have all now become loyal customers. I look forward to many more years of friendly professional appointments

Sarah Trevett

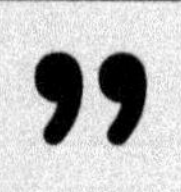

6. Use ingredient and Nutrition Facts labels to discover what various foods contain so that you can make healthier choices.
7. Avoid or minimize foods that are high in solid fats and added sugar. Limit processed meats, cakes, biscuits, sweets, and ice cream.
8. Eat at home more often so you can control what you are eating. If you eat out, choose healthier options such as baked potato instead of french fries.[85]

BALANCED DIET—IS THE PYRAMID STILL APPLICABLE?

"You don't have to eat less; you just have to eat right."
~Unknown

The familiar food pyramid introduced in 1991 was supposed to be our nutrition guide. However, many people found the pyramid to be confusing. And it didn't help us to plan a healthy diet, one meal at a time. Most importantly, nutrition has to be personalized for each individual because each of us is unique.

So, in May 2011, the USDA finally discarded the pyramid concept in favour of a plate. Their "MyPyramid" website was also revamped and redirected to a new online site: www.ChooseMyPlate.gov.

While the basic nutritional guidelines for Americans remain the same, the old pyramid and the USDA Plate have a few significant differences:

85 https://www.choosemyplate.gov/ten-tips-make-better-food-choices

I am extremely satisfied and overwhelmed with the results I have seen from the Chiropractic care at AVID Clinic.

When I came for my initial check-up I was lacking energy in my every day life and was not able to digest food properly.

Trishul Vadi the lead Chiropractor was very caring and empathetic towards my concerns & needs as he gave me a full thorough examination.

I underwent a full treatment plan and as the weeks went by I noticed an improvement in my sleep and my food started to digest more efficiently resulting in an improvement in my day to day enthusiasm.

I am now 1000% better than before having the treatment and definitely recommend AVID Clinic to everyone!

Thank you so much AVID Clinic :)

Gabriel Coniah

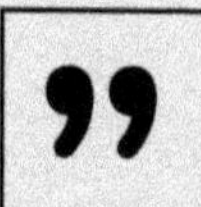

- The food pyramid was dominated by grains, which filled in the largest spot at the bottom of the pyramid. The Plate version reserves only one quadrant for grains (mainly whole grains) and reserves half the plate for fruits and vegetables, more than any other food group. This is a major improvement since most of us don't eat enough vegetables and fruits
- Fats, oils and sugars appeared on the old pyramid in small quantities with the message to eat these foods rarely or in small amounts. These don't show up anywhere on the Plate, though dietary fat is essential for optimal health. However, the ChooseMyPlate.gov site provides in-depth information about fats, oils and added sugars.
- The food guide pyramid told you how many servings of each food group to consume each day. The Plate does not mention how many servings you should eat of any food group. The lack of serving sizes makes the Plate simpler to implement and understand than the pyramid. And the ChooseMyPlate.gov site allows you to enter your personal data and get an individualized eating plan.
- The pyramid featured only food groups; however, the plate adds protein as one of the elements. Protein is a nutrient found in various foods, not an actual food group. It seems out of place along with fruits (food), vegetables (food), grains (food), and milk (food). Protein seems to be a simplification of the meat, beans, nuts, and legumes food group. The USDA says that "protein" means a variety of sources such as meat, eggs, dairy, nuts, seeds, beans, soy, etc.

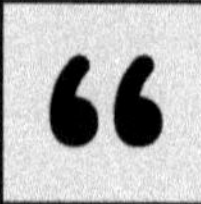

Fantastic team. The service is excellent. Always helpful and ready to listen to whatever queries you have. I have made good progress since I started my treatment. Will recommend them to anyone with back problems any day.

Naana Teye

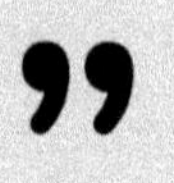

The Plate as an icon is easier to understand than the pyramid. You can look at it once and easily remember what it conveys, and which food groups it includes. You can stick the Choose My Plate symbol on your kitchen wall as a reference guide. The aim is to match your dinner plate with the four quadrants in the Plate for a balanced and nutritious meal.[86]

KETOGENIC DIET

"Healthy eating is a way of life, so it's important to establish routines that are simple, realistic, and ultimately liveable."
~Horace

A ketogenic or keto diet is a diet that causes the body to release ketones into the bloodstream.

Blood sugar, which comes from carbohydrates, is the body's main source of energy. In the absence of blood sugar, we start breaking down stored fat into molecules called ketone bodies using a process called ketosis. Once we reach ketosis, most cells will use ketone bodies to generate energy until we start eating carbohydrates again.

The shift, from using circulating glucose to breaking down stored fat as a source of energy, usually happens over two to four days of eating fewer than 20 to 50 grams of carbohydrates per day.

Because it lacks carbohydrates, a ketogenic diet is rich in proteins and fats. It typically includes plenty of meats, eggs, processed meats, sausages, cheeses, fish, nuts, butter, oils, seeds, and fibrous vegetables. Because it is so restrictive, it is really hard to follow over the long run.

86 https://www.sparkpeople.com/resource/nutrition_articles.asp?id=425

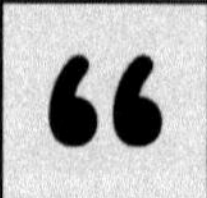

Always amazingly friendly and professional service. Would recommend AVID Clinic to everyone!

Beth Parrott

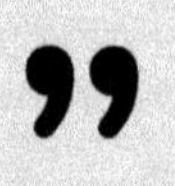

Carbohydrates normally account for at least 50% of the typical American diet. One of the main criticisms of this diet is that many people tend to eat too much protein and poor-quality fats from processed foods, with very few fruits and vegetables. Patients with kidney disease need to be cautious because this diet could worsen their condition.

Is a ketogenic diet healthy?

Weight loss is the primary reason my patients use the ketogenic diet. Previous research shows good evidence of a faster weight loss when patients go on a ketogenic or very low carbohydrate diet compared to participants on a more traditional low-fat diet, or even a Mediterranean diet. However, that difference in weight loss seems to disappear over time.

A ketogenic diet also has been shown to improve blood sugar control for patients with type 2 diabetes, in the short term. However, there is no long-term research analysing its long-term effects on diabetes and high cholesterol.

Though a ketogenic diet may accelerate weight loss, it's hard to follow and has unhealthy foods such as red meat and dairy. Its long-term effects are not well known, probably because it's so hard to follow it for a long time! Such yo-yo diets that lead to rapid weight loss fluctuation are associated with increased mortality. A balanced plant-based diet comprising colourful fruits and vegetables, whole grains, nuts, seeds, olive oil, fish and lean meats seems to be a better option than a keto diet.[87]

87 https://www.health.harvard.edu/blog/ketogenic-diet-is-the-ultimate-low-carb-diet-good-for-you-2017072712089

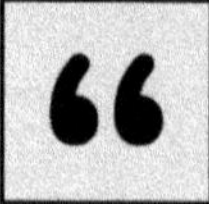

I have been using AVID for over a year, firstly when I had sciatica which is the most excruciating illness every I have experienced. After a few months AVID Clinic had cleared this awful pain. I still go regularly for back, knee, foot problems and would highly recommend the AVID Clinic.

Geoff Tookey

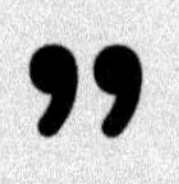

PESCATARIAN DIET

"Every time you eat is an opportunity to nourish your body."
~Unknown

A pescatarian or pesco-vegetarian diet is a vegetarian diet that also includes fish as an additional protein source. A pescatarian diet has many of the benefits of a plant-based diet, including reduced inflammation and lower risk of diabetes and heart disease.

A pescatarian diet also helps to round out many of the nutritional deficiencies that can be present in a typical vegetarian diet, because fatty seafood contains vitamin D and beneficial omega-3 fatty acids. Seafood also contains iron, calcium and vitamin B12, which can be lacking in many vegetarian diets.

One of the biggest disadvantages of a pescatarian diet is that some types of fish can be high in mercury, a neurotoxin that can cause muscle weakness, loss of peripheral vision, impaired fine motor skills, tremors, headaches, insomnia and emotional changes. Smaller fish tend to have much less mercury content than larger fish, so they're safer to eat.

By combining data from the U.S. Food and Drug Administration and the U.S. Environmental Protection Agency, the National Resource Defense Council grouped fish into four categories based on their mercury content:

- **least mercury** (eat at will): anchovies, herring, North Atlantic mackerel, pollock, sardines, shrimp, freshwater trout, squid, clams, crayfish and catfish.

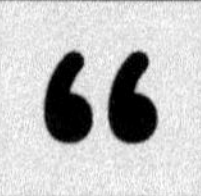

I have been coming to AVID Clinic with my mother for over 10 years and have never been anywhere else. The Clinic is clean, the staff are all wonderful and the treatments are so varied. Highly recommended!

Sarah Moore

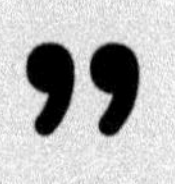

- **moderate mercury** (eat six or fewer servings per month): carp, cod, bass, mahi-mahi, lobster, snapper, freshwater perch, and skipjack or canned chunk light tuna.
- **high mercury** (three servings or less per month): halibut, ocean perch, Chilean sea bass, albacore or yellowfin tuna, and Spanish mackerel.
- **highest mercury** (avoid eating these fish): bluefish, grouper, king mackerel, marlin, swordfish, bigeye and ahi tuna, shark and orange roughy.[88]

Other disadvantages of a pescatarian diet include ethical questions about fish farming and wild harvesting practices such as the use of antibiotics, overfishing, and bycatch.[89]

PALEO DIET

"Health is a relationship between you and your body."
~Terri Guillemets

A paleo diet is based on foods similar to what might have been eaten during the Palaeolithic era, which dates from approximately 2.5 million to 10,000 years ago. Other names for a paleo diet are Palaeolithic diet, Stone Age diet, hunter-gatherer diet and caveman diet. A paleo diet comprises foods that could be obtained by hunting and gathering in the past, such as lean meat, fish, fruits, vegetables, nuts and seeds. A paleo diet limits foods like dairy products, legumes and grains that became common when farming emerged about 10,000 years ago.

88 https://www.nrdc.org/stories/smart-seafood-buying-guide
89 https://www.livestrong.com/article/399500-the-disadvantages-of-a-pescetarian-diet/

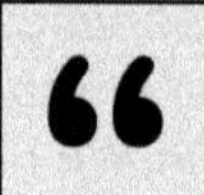

Excellent service and very friendly. As a dentist I felt it was important to look after my posture and back for my career and found Trishul and Komal to be fantastic for preventative care. Five years later I'm still here.

Dr Roy Woodhoo

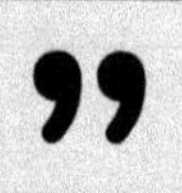

The aim of a paleo diet is to return to a way of eating that's more like what early humans ate. It is claimed to help you to lose weight and maintain a healthy weight.

Paleo diets follow these general guidelines:

- **Eat:** fruits, vegetables, nuts, seeds, lean meat, especially grass-fed animals or wild game, fish, oils from fruits and nuts like olive oil or walnut oil
- **Avoid:** grains like wheat, oats and barley, legumes like beans, lentils, peanuts and peas, dairy products, sugar, salt, potatoes, and highly processed foods in general

The diet also recommends drinking only water and being physically active every day.

Several randomized Clinical trials have compared the paleo diet to other diets such as the Mediterranean Diet. A paleo diet may provide benefits such as

- more weight loss
- improved glucose tolerance
- better blood pressure control
- lower triglycerides
- better appetite management

However, longer trials are needed to understand the long-term health benefits and possible risks of a paleo diet.

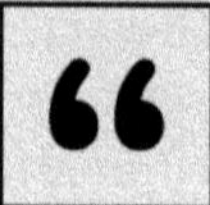

First class service, Trishul Vadi is always happy to help with outstanding advice...

Paul Freemantle

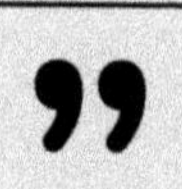

Dietary concerns

A paleo diet is rich in vegetables, fruits and nuts. However, it excludes whole grains and legumes, which are good sources of fibre, vitamins and other nutrients. It also excludes dairy products, which are good sources of protein and calcium.

These foods are more affordable and accessible than foods such as wild game, grass-fed animals and nuts. So a paleo diet may be too expensive for some people.

You might be able to achieve better health benefits as a Paleo diet by eating a balanced, healthy diet that includes whole grains and legumes.[90]

POOP AS AN INDICATOR OF HEALTH

"If you can't pronounce it, don't eat it."
~Michael Pollan

Poop (faeces) is mostly undigested food, proteins, bacteria, salts, and other substances that are produced and released by intestines. Healthy poop has a wide range of variations.[91]

The Bristol Stool Scale is an indicator of the different types of poops. It's broken up into seven categories based on a 2,000-person study.

90 https://www.mayoClinic.org/healthy-lifestyle/nutrition-and-healthy-eating/in-depth/paleo-diet/art-20111182
91 https://www.healthline.com/health/digestive-health/types-of-poop

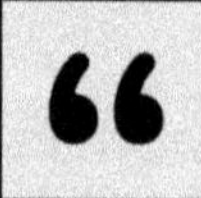

A thoroughly professional assessment and treatment. I used to be in regular neck and back pain. Now with all AVID's help and treatments this is a thing of the past.

Thoroughly recommend.

Alan Willingale

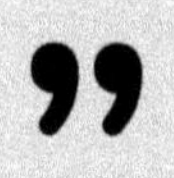

Type	Appearance	Indicates
Type 1	Hard and separate little lumps that look like nuts and are hard to pass	These little pellets typically mean you're constipated. It shouldn't happen frequently.
Type 2	Log-shaped but lumpy	Here we have another sign of constipation that, again, shouldn't happen frequently.
Type 3	Log-shaped with some cracks on the surface	This is the gold standard of poop, especially if it's somewhat soft and easy to pass.
Type 4	Smooth and snake-like	Doctors also consider this a normal poop that should happen every one to three days.
Type 5	These are small, like the first ones, but soft and easy to pass. The blobs also have clear cut edges.	This type of poop means you are lacking fibre and should find ways to add some to your diet through cereal or vegetables.
Type 6	Fluffy and mushy with ragged edges.	This too-soft consistency could be a sign of mild diarrhoea. Try drinking more water and fruit juice to help improve this.
Type 7	Completely watery with no solid pieces.	In other words, you've got diarrhoea. This means your stool moved through your bowels very quickly and didn't form into a healthy poop.[92]

92 https://continence.org.au/pages/bristol-stool-chart.html

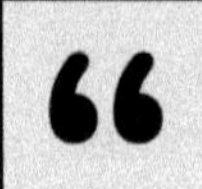

This is a little sanctuary in West Wickham. Fabulous family run team and I can't recommend enough.

Sarah Alpert

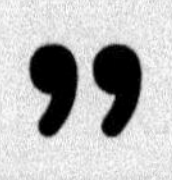

Poop colour: Poop comes in a range of colours. All shades of brown and even green are considered normal. Stool colour is influenced by what you eat as well as by the amount of bile in your stool. (Bile is a yellow-green fluid that digests fats.) Seek prompt medical attention if your poop is bright red or black because it may indicate the presence of blood.

Stool quality	**What it may mean**	**Possible dietary causes**
Green	Food may be moving through the large intestine too quickly, such as due to diarrhoea. As a result, bile doesn't have time to break down completely.	Green leafy vegetables, green food colouring, such as in flavoured drink mixes or ice pops, iron supplements.
Light-coloured, white or clay-coloured	A lack of bile in stool. This may indicate a bile duct obstruction.	Certain medications, such as large doses of bismuth subsalicylate (Kaopectate, Pepto-Bismol) and other anti-diarrheal drugs.
Yellow, greasy, foul-smelling	Excess fat in the stool, such as due to a malabsorption disorder, for example, celiac disease.	Sometimes the protein gluten, such as in bread and cereals. See a doctor for evaluation.
Black	Bleeding in the upper gastrointestinal tract, such as the stomach.	Iron supplements, bismuth subsalicylate (Kaopectate, Pepto-Bismol), black liquorice.
Bright red	Bleeding in the lower intestinal tract, such as the large intestine or rectum, often from haemorrhoids.	Red food colouring, beets, cranberries, tomato juice or soup, red gelatin or drink mixes.[93]

93 https://www.mayoClinic.org/stool-color/expert-answers/faq-20058080

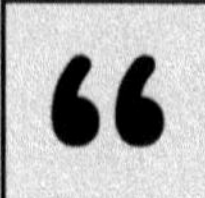

I've been coming to AVID for 10 years now, they are so professional, kind and friendly.

Lucy Ede

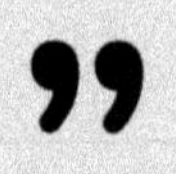

BEST RECOMMENDATIONS

"Moderation. Small helpings. Sample a little bit of everything. These are the secrets of happiness and good health." ~Julia Child

Most diets, including raw food, paleo and keto, aren't sustainable over a long period because of individual lifestyle, activity level, food preferences, lack of support, and so on.

Your long-term health results are dependent on your behaviour not on your diet. For a healthy body and a healthy body weight, you have to develop consistent, sustainable daily habits. For example, instead of eating 800 calories one day and then eating 3,000 calories the next day, aim to eat just above the amount you can stick with, and reduce it in small amounts over time, if needed. Aim for progress in small increments (kaizen).

Other healthy strategies you can adopt, while enjoying the foods you love:

- eat slowly and mindfully
- eat until you're 80% full
- eat greater amounts of minimally processed foods
- eat more fibre and protein
- get more high-quality sleep
- move throughout the day and minimize immobility
- exercise regularly to improve your strength, endurance, flexibility and balance
- take steps to reduce stress and build resilience (meditation)
- spend quality time with family and friends[94]

94 https://www.precisionnutrition.com/calories-in-calories-out

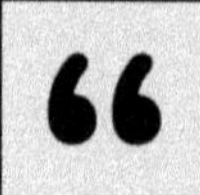

I came to AVID Clinic in extreme pain and could hardly move. Brilliant consultation resulting in being pain free and able to work and continue my fitness regime. Highly recommend AVID for chiropractic treatment.

Nakita Ross

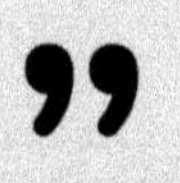

TIME-THE ENIGMA OF LIFE

"Healing is an art. It takes time. It takes practice.
It takes love."
~Maza Dohta

"It's up to you to protect and maintain your body's innate capacity for health and healing by making the right choices in how you live."
~Andrew Weil

HEALING TAKES TIME

Good health takes time and commitment. Your symptoms didn't develop overnight. They are usually a gradual but progressive buildup of toxicity and physical changes.

However, this is the age of instant gratification. Most of us tend to be impatient and want instant relief. Unfortunately, instant relief is not healing. Instant relief masks our symptoms without restoring the body to its natural healthy state.

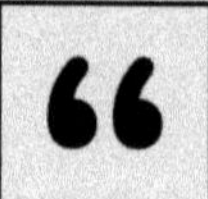

Very friendly staff and I have had a really good treatment with Trishul all along. Would definitely recommend

Ilhan Akyurek

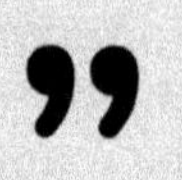

For example, most drugs give instant relief by masking our symptoms. So you have to keep taking them to continue to get relief. However, when we discontinue the drug, the symptoms return almost immediately. Ideally, the drug should correct the problem so that we can stop taking the drug after a reasonable period. Usually, that is not the case.

For example, have you ever known anyone whose anti-diabetes medications healed them of diabetes so they could discontinue the drug? How about high blood pressure? Migraine? Heart disease? Usually, we have to take them lifelong because medications can control these disorders but cannot reverse or cure them.

On the other hand, a nutritional and lifestyle program addresses the real root causes of your illness. If you stay on the program for the prescribed duration, you get better and regain your health.

Real Healing takes time. It may take several months to fully recover from a chronic health problem. It may even take several years to completely overcome a degenerative condition. However, it doesn't take that long to see improvement. Just as a seed sprouts and begins to grow long before the plant matures fully, you can see the signs that your health is improving long before you are completely healed.

So, if a particular therapy doesn't bring about any improvement at all within a reasonable period, you may need to review your options.

What is a reasonable amount of time for healing?

The time you take to heal depends on many factors such as the nature of the disorder, your immunity, the severity and duration of the illness, etc. With acute illness, you should see some improvement within a day or two. Chronic illnesses may take a few days to improve. Degenerative illnesses may take even longer, especially if they involve organs, bones and joints.

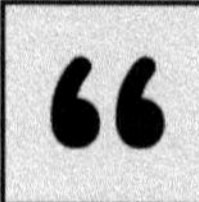

The staff are lovely and friendly and always make you feel very welcome and comfortable. My back feels great.

Abigail Smith

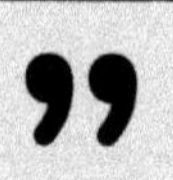

Improvement means you should feel better. The true test of any therapy is how it affects your body and mind. Do you feel more energetic? Is your sense of well-being improving? Are you feeling more alive and healthy? You need to learn to listen to your own body and trust what it is telling you.

When the cause of your disease is removed, you will notice that your symptoms are decreasing, and your energy levels are increasing. On the contrary, if the body cannot eliminate the root cause of your illness, it overpowers your body's defensive mechanisms. This leads to stagnation, lower energy levels and progressive weakening of our organ systems.

There are two reasons for the failure in healing:

- The immunity of your body was too weak to resist the irritant and overcome it. That's the reason why restoring your immunity and health is the foundation of healthcare. The stronger your immunity, the more easily it will defend your health.
- Your immune response is suppressed by pain killers and other medications. Symptoms, such as fever, runny nose, sneezing, diarrhoea, coughing, etc. are ways to eliminate irritants. The instant relief of symptoms by medications interferes with these natural body responses. They interfere with natural body processes. When you take these medications, your body is not really cured. The problem is suppressed and turns into a chronic or degenerative disease.[95]

95 https://www.webnat.com/articles/Healing.asp

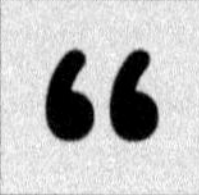

This is a wonderful practice and in the space of nine months has restored my mobility and general sense of well being. I am a retired GP. They think of everything and their approach is deeply holistic and empathic. I would have no hesitation in recommending all of them to my colleagues...

Dr James Pitt-Payne

Retired GP & Psychotherapist

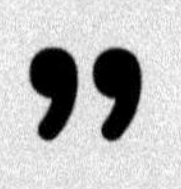

The vast number of challenges our body can face, all have different responses, and every person's response is unique. What we do know is that true healing and correction are not instantaneous (and if they were, they would be unsustainable); time is the KEY to making true change. Small, specific, sustained changes bring about the biggest and sustainable change – be patient with your body, it certainly is patient with you.

Patients often say it is their age that results in them feeling and presenting the way that they are, but is this necessarily true and does age affect healing? Is age associated with longer healing times? Let's have a look.

WHY DOES THE BODY AGE, AND HOW DOES IT AGE?

Aging is a complex process that affects different people and even different organs in diverse ways. No single process can explain all the changes caused by aging. It's due to the interaction of many lifelong influences, including heredity, environment, diet, exercise, past illnesses, genes, lifestyle, and many other factors.

The cause and mechanism of aging are not clear. It could be a predetermined process controlled by genes or it could be due to long-term injuries caused by ultraviolet light or the by-products of metabolism such as free radicals.

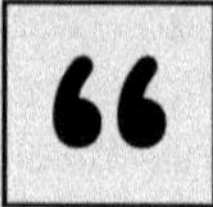

This Clinic has a lateral approach enabling all types of personalities to gain expertise offered. I personally have been able to carry out normal pursuits with less pain than I had before. I will continue to attend this Clinic as I feel the ongoing benefits are paramount.

Janice Redway

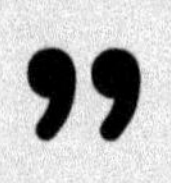

Each person ages differently. Although some changes always occur with aging, they occur at different rates and to different extents. Some systems begin aging as early as age 30. Other aging processes are not common until much later in life. There is no way to predict exactly how you will age.[96]

IS DEGENERATION ASSOCIATED WITH AGE?

Our bodies change with age because of changes in individual cells and organs. These changes result in changes in function and appearance. Some age-related functional changes are as follows:

- **Mental function**
- **Difficulty learning new material:** The number of receptors on nerve cells may decrease. Thus, the brain does not send or process impulse as well or as quickly.
- **Physical activity**
- **Unsteadiness or loss of balance:** Structures in the inner ear that help with balance stiffen and deteriorate slightly. The part of the brain that controls balance (cerebellum) may degenerate.
- **Dizziness or light-headedness when standing:** The heart does not pump enough blood to the head because the heart is less able to respond to changes in position. The blood vessels do not constrict enough to maintain normal blood pressure when a person stands.

96 https://medlineplus.gov/ency/article/004012.htm

Friendly and knowledgeable, I've been a client for years and would highly recommend. The new premises are fantastic and just add to the feeling of being cared for professionally.

Gill Chamberlain

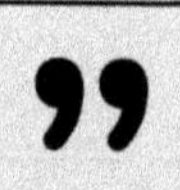

- **Loss of muscle strength:** The number and size of muscle fibres decrease. The body produces less growth hormone (and less testosterone in men).
- **Difficulty moving and less flexibility:** Less joint fluid is produced. Muscle tissue is lost, decreasing strength and making muscles stiffer.
- **Difficulty exercising strenuously:** The heart cannot keep up with the demand for more blood during exercise. The lungs cannot keep up with the demand for oxygen during exercise.
- **The senses**
- **Need for reading glasses:** The lens of the eye stiffens, making focusing on close objects more difficult.
- **Difficulty seeing in dim light:** The retina of the eye becomes less sensitive to light. The lens of the eye becomes less transparent.
- **Difficulty adjusting to changes in light levels:** The pupils react more slowly to changes in light.
- **Dry eyes:** The number of cells that produce fluids to lubricate the eyes decreases. The tear glands produce fewer tears.
- **Loss of hearing:** Age-related hearing loss (presbycusis) develops.
- **Loss of taste:** Taste buds become less sensitive.
- **Dry mouth:** Less saliva is produced.

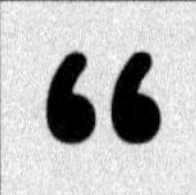

We have had a wonderful experience at AVID Clinic. We always receive a warm, friendly and personal welcome on arrival.

My son is receiving treatment and Trishul has gone out of their way to ensure he understands what they are doing, why they are doing it and what he can expect - plus they tell great stories!!!

Suzanne St Clair

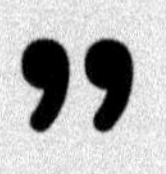

- **Eating problems**
- **Difficulty swallowing:** The mouth is dry. People may not chew food enough because teeth are missing or dentures do not fit well.
- **Disinterest in eating:** Taste and smell decreases, making food less appetizing.
- **Skin and hair**
- **Wrinkles:** The fat layer under the skin thins.
- **Dry skin:** Glands in the skin produce less oil.
- **Bruises:** Blood vessels in the skin become more fragile.
- **Decreased sensation:** The number of nerve endings in the skin decreases.
- **Gray or white hair:** The hair follicles produce less pigment (melanin).
- **Thinning or loss of hair:** Some hair follicles stop producing new hair.
- **Sexual function**
- **Dryness of the vagina:** Less oestrogen is produced.
- **Erections that do not last as long, are less rigid, or take more time:** Less testosterone is produced. Blood flow to the penis decreases.[97]

However, there is no need to feel overly depressed or anxious. Most of the significant age-related health issues can be minimized by a healthy lifestyle and a positive attitude. As Mark Twain said, "Age is an issue of mind over matter. If you don't mind, it doesn't matter." He also said, "Wrinkles should merely indicate where smiles have been."

97 https://www.merckmanuals.com/home/older-people%E2%80%99s-health-issues/the-aging-body/changes-in-the-body-with-aging

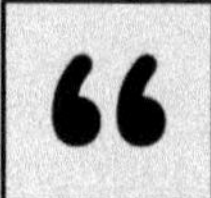

I have seen Trishul both as a patient and in a professional capacity for a number of years. Throughout this time I have found him to be very caring & professional and certainly would highly recommend him to any one requiring treatment.

Nigel Jackson

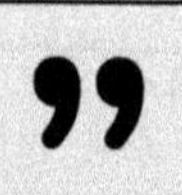

AGE-RELATED LOSS OF FLEXIBILITY

In healthy older adults aged 55 to 85 years, age-related loss of flexibility appears to be small such that the normal loss of joint range of motion is unlikely to neither affect daily functions nor cause disability.[98]

Many age-related changes including declines in flexibility are caused by disuse and a sedentary lifestyle. Men are more likely to have decreased flexibility than women.

Exercise, stretching, yoga, and manual therapy can reverse many many age-related changes including decreased flexibility. However, exercise needs to be approached cautiously with long warm-ups, long cool-downs and adequate recovery in order to prevent injury, especially if you've been sedentary. It is best to seek the guidance of a manual therapist or physical trainer.[99]

Time, movement, hydration, balanced nutrition and a positive mindset are all vital in healing; and all need to be addressed when proactively working towards health. Be patient and concerted in your efforts, it really is that simple.

---

98 https://www.hindawi.com/journals/jar/2013/743843/

99 https://www.naturalathleteClinic.com/blogs/natural-athlete-solutions/preventing-age-related-declines-in-flexibility

I had really bad back problems before finding these guys and they have helped me back to normal, they are very professional and the staff are very helpful highly recommend to anyone.

Jonathan Smith

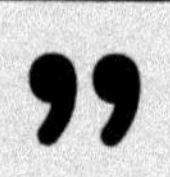

09

HYDRATE-THE ELIXIR OF LIFE

"You are 87% water; the other 13% keeps you from drowning."
~P. E. Morris

"Drinking water is like washing out your insides. The water will cleanse the system, fill you up, decrease your caloric load and improve the function of all your tissues."
~Kevin R. Stone

Good hydration is vital for good health.

Water makes up about two thirds of your body and about 73% of your brain.[100] Every organ in your body needs water to function properly. You need water to maintain your body temperature, get rid of waste, lubricate your joints and for general good health.[101] Good hydration has been shown to reduce the risk of many health disorders such as constipation, hypertension, kidney stones, urinary tract infections, and exercise asthma.[102]

100 Mitchell HH et al. (1945) The chemical composition of the adult human body and its bearing on the biochemistry of growth. Journal of Biological Chemistry 158(3): 625-37

101 https://www.ncbi.nlm.nih.gov/pubmed/19724292

102 https://www.ncbi.nlm.nih.gov/pubmed/16028566

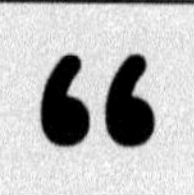

I have been coming to the AVID Clinic for a number of years and can't recommend them enough. A family run Clinic extremely professional and friendly. The chiropractic services have been so helpful in alleviating and managing my ailments. The beauty services are fantastic too. Highly recommend

Shipra Sharma

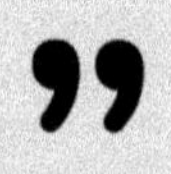

HOW MUCH WATER DO YOU NEED?

Water is essential for the maintenance of normal physical and cognitive functions and normal thermo-regulation.[103] Based on the European Food Safety Authority's scientific estimation of adequate water intake, men should aim for a total water intake of 2.5 litres per day whereas women should aim for a total water intake of 2 litres per day. Ideally, 70-80% of this should come from drinks and 20-30% from foods.[104]

Average Water Input=2.5 litres	**Average Water Output=2.5 litres**
Water in fluids: 1.5 litres	Urine: 1.6 litres
Water in food: 0.7 litres	Sweat: 0.45 litres
Metabolic water: 0.3 litres	Breathing: 0.35 litres
	Faeces: 0.2 litres
Total: 2.5 litres	**Total: 2.5 litres**

Water balance in sedentary adults living in temperate climate[105]

Usually, the contribution of food to total dietary fluid intake is 20–30%, whereas 70–80% is provided by drinks. This relationship is not fixed and depends on the type of drinks and the choice of foods. Foods have a wide range of water content (from less than 40% to more than 80%).

103 EFSA (2011) Scientific Opinion on the substantiation of health claims related to water and maintenance of normal physical and cognitive functions (ID 1102, 1209, 1294, 1331), maintenance of normal thermoregulation (ID 1208) and "basic requirement of all living things" (ID 1207) pursuant to Article 13(1) of Regulation (EC) No 1924/2006. EFSA Journal 9(4):2075

104 EFSA (2010) Scientific Opinion on Dietary Reference Values for water. EFSA Journal 8(3):1459

105 https://www.ncbi.nlm.nih.gov/pubmed/19724292

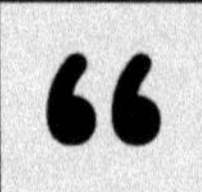

Lovely environment and professional throughout. Wasn't sure my back would feel better but Trishul managed to fix it. Feeling like new :)

Xavier Wing Hing

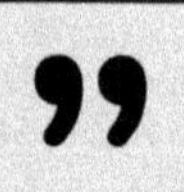

Your water requirement changes throughout the day. Ideally, your water intake should equal your water requirement over 24 hours.[106]

If water intake is less than our requirement, we become dehydrated. This is more likely in hot and dry conditions, especially if we have limited access to water and lose more water than usual through excessive sweating, diarrhoea or vomiting.

Mild dehydration may occur when we lose about 1-2 percent of our body weight. Some common symptoms of mild to moderate dehydration include thirst, dark-coloured urine, less frequent urination, fatigue, dizziness, constipation, and confusion.[107]

DIFFERENT FORMS OF FLUIDS

Water: Science has proved the truth of this ancient Slovakian proverb, "Pure water is the world's first and foremost medicine." Water has zero calories and is the best way to quench your thirst. Drink tap water. You don't need to drink bottled water; tap water is good enough. However, you may need to filter it before drinking. To make water more refreshing, add a slice of lemon or lime.

Tea and coffee: You should limit your daily caffeine intake to about 400 mg, which is equal to 750 ml of black coffee (3 cups) or 1 litre of black tea per day (4 cups). If you are pregnant, limit your caffeine intake to 500 ml of coffee (2 cups) or 750 ml of tea (3 cups). Drink herbal tea or decaffeinated coffee or tea if you want to have more than the recommended amount of caffeinated drinks. Avoid specialty coffees and teas because they are high in sugar.

106 https://www.ncbi.nlm.nih.gov/pmc/articles/PMC4207053/
107 https://www.mayoClinic.org/diseases-conditions/dehydration/symptoms-causes/syc-20354086

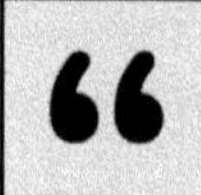

Fixed my back after 12 years of manual labour and an extremely welcoming community

Lee Millward

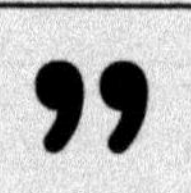

Fruit and vegetable juice: Limit your intake of fruit juices since they are high in calories and low in fibre. Eat the fruit instead. Make sure you choose 100% real fruit juice. Avoid fruit drinks, cocktails or punches as they have added sugar and few nutrients.

Fizzy drinks: Avoid these drinks because they are high in calories, sugar and chemicals. Some fizzy drinks like colas may also contain caffeine. Diet fizzy drinks are calorie and sugar free but may have caffeine, artificial sweeteners and other chemicals.

Sports drinks: Commercial sports drinks are usually not needed to keep hydrated when you exercise. Many of them contain ingredients that are unhealthy. Water and a healthy diet can replace water and minerals lost during exercise.[108]

Alcohol: Minimize alcoholic drinks. The immediate effects of cutting down alcohol include feeling better in the morning, being less tired during the day, better-looking skin, feeling more energetic, and better weight management. Long-term benefits include improved mood, sleep, judgement, memory, immunity, behaviour, and overall health.[109] The next time you are tempted to drink with friends, remember this wise Chinese proverb: "With true friends...even water drunk together is sweet enough."

---

108 https://www.dietitians.ca/getattachment/becace49-3bad-4754-ac94-f31c3f04fed0/FACTSHEET-Guidelines-for-staying-hydrated.pdf.aspx

109 https://www.nhs.uk/live-well/alcohol-support/tips-on-cutting-down-alcohol/

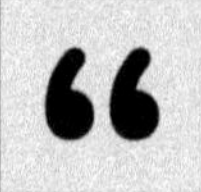

Words can not explain how good the AVID Clinic have helped me with my lower back pain. From a friendly smile at reception to a cheerful hello from Trishul highly recommendable!

Paul Hooper

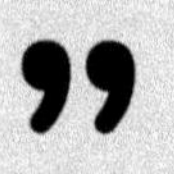

DEHYDRATION IN THE UK

A survey carried out by the Royal National Lifeboat Institution showed that 89% of the population is not drinking enough water to maintain healthy hydration levels. Men are less hydrated than women: 20% of men drink no water at all during the day compared with 13% of women. The elderly are less hydrated: 25% of those over 55 stated that they drink no water during the day compared with 7% of those aged 25-34.[110]

TOP TIPS FOR HEALTHY HYDRATION

1. Drink water. It is the best way to hydrate as it has no calories, sugar or artificial chemicals. Heed these words of Thoreau, "Water is the only drink for a wise man."
2. Choose food with high water content such as soups, stews, vegetables, and fruits to increase your overall daily water intake.
3. Sip water regularly throughout the day because hydration levels fluctuate throughout the day.
4. Drink more water when you exercise or spend time in hot and dry environments.
5. Make sure to carry water with you, especially when you are travelling. Keep water nearby when you are at work, at school or playing.
6. Make sure you are drinking pure water. Use a water filter if necessary.
7. Avoid or minimize unhealthy drinks such as soft drinks, caffeinated drinks and alcohol.[111]

110 https://www.naturalhydrationcouncil.org.uk/press/how-hydrated-is-britain/

111 Dr Emma Derbyshire PhD, National Hydration Council, The Essential Guide to Hydration

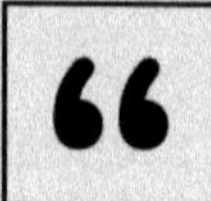

Good work done for my back. Great people looking after me.

Doru Merauta

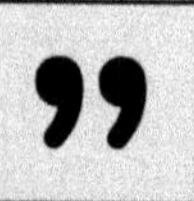

FINAL TIP – LISTEN TO YOUR BODY

- **Check your thirst:** If you are thirsty or have a dry mouth, you may not be drinking enough water. Remember that when you are thirsty, you are already somewhat dehydrated. Aim to drink fluids often throughout the day.
- **Check your urine:** If your urine is a dark yellow colour and has a strong smell, you may not be getting enough fluids. Urine that is light yellow or clear in colour usually means that you are drinking enough fluids. The amount of urine you make can also be a sign of your hydration status. If you do not make much urine throughout the day and it is dark in colour, you need more fluids.
- **Check your mood:** If you feel tired, are not able to focus or have headaches, these could be signs that you are dehydrated.[112]

112 https://www.unlockfood.ca/en/Articles/Water/Facts-on-Fluids-How-to-Stay-Hydrated.aspx

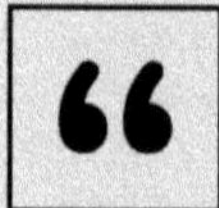

I have been coming to AVID Clinic for many years and have recommended them to my friends and family. They provide an excellent service and my problems have got a lot better.

Pauline Andrews

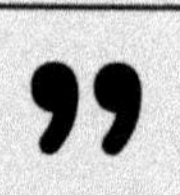

10

PARTING WORDS

"Health is the new wealth. We will still define success by how nice our house is or the zip code we live in. But going forward, health is going to become increasingly synonymous with social status. Health will be a currency of its own. You cannot necessarily buy health, but you will know how to earn it, and you earn it every day of your life."
~Henry Loubet, CEO, Bohemia Health

"Never doubt that a small group of thoughtful, committed citizens can change the world; indeed, it's the only thing that ever has."
~Margaret Mead

Congratulations on finishing the book! Whether you read every page or read the chapters that were of interest to you, you took the first step. You rock!

Nine out of ten people who purchase books don't finish them. That's why Groucho Marx said, 'From the moment I picked up your book until I put it down, I was convulsed with laughter. Some day I intend reading it.'

You are in the tiny minority of people who have decided to take charge of your health and seek information and help. That is the first right step.

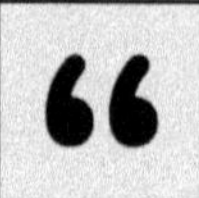

I came to the Clinic for help with weakness in my knee resulting from a longstanding injury. They set me a course of osteopathic treatment and exercises which helped realign my spinal column and strengthen the muscles around my knee. The difference in my stature and the strength in the muscles around my knees was quickly noticeable. I will be continue the exercises and visits to the Clinic to maintain the correct position of my spinal frame.

Maggie Jackson

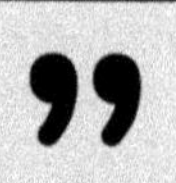

As already explained, the vital principles that will help you to achieve your health goals are:

H – Hydrate

E – Exercise

A – AVIDttitude Shift

L – Living Food

T – Time

H – Happiness

The most important takeaway from this book is that you have to take responsibility for your own health by nurturing your body and mind. And that starts with making the right choices.

The journey of a thousand miles begins with the first step. Choose one baby step that you can do right now. Do a single push-up or squat. Or drink a glass of water. Or spend some quality time with your family. Whatever it is, stop reading and do it right now.

One final caveat: Each one of us is different with individual health issues determined by our age, gender, genes, environment, emotions, and past illnesses. Please consult your health professional before making any major decision that may affect your health.

I hope this book was helpful to you. If you have any questions or comments, please contact us at AVIDClinic.co.uk or 020 8777 4343. We would love to hear from you.

All the best for your onward journey to a happy, healthy and harmonious life!

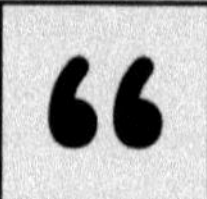

Wonderful has helped my shoulder so much, so thank you.

Carol Rogers

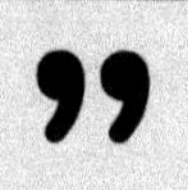

Health & Happiness

Dr Trishul Vadi

BOst, MChiro, MMCA, MCO, PG Cert HE

Clinic Director, Osteopath and Doctor of Chiropractic at AVID Clinic

P.S.

"Happily ever after is not a fairy tale—it's a choice."
~Fawn Weaver

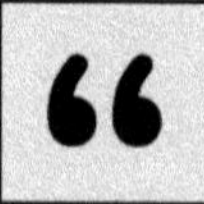

AVID Clinic is a great place to come for adjustments. The people are friendly and really make you feel welcome and like part of the family. I would definitely recommend coming to AVID!

Dhuran Modha

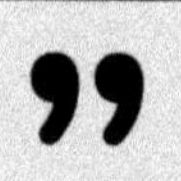

11

AVID CLINIC

AVID Clinic has been providing services to South London since 1995. We have grown from strength to strength and are recognised as one of UK's leading Clinics.

It is our intention to provide the best quality care to all by serving and educating our thriving community on health, strength and wellness.

We believe in a life that is lived naturally, and to its optimum expression – thank you for choosing us to guide you on your journey to your best life.

Since the first review I made which was when I had first visited AVID Clinic for my consultation I have now had 2 'practical' appointments, where treatment has been given in the form of some very much needed pushing, rubbing, 'popping' and cracking of bones etc - it's nowhere near as bad as that makes it sound, if anything it has actually given me a spring in my step after just 2 treatments. I was open-minded when I went there and the service seemed great, hence the initial review. Since I have started treatment though I have to say that my experience has gone from excellent to outstanding and the overall service from the welcoming with herbal teas to the actual treatment and after-care is absolutely second to none. Trishul is one of the most knowledgeable and straight forward practitioners I have ever come across in any form of treatments and practices, he is also very personable and thorough in everything he does and whilst some of the treatments are short in time he never clock watches and if you have questions or need more attention on anything, he is always willing to go that extra mile and give you all the time he can. I also love that this is very much a family business and from start to finish everything about it has had that family feel yet has been a beacon of professionalism as well, which is often difficult to get that balance but AVID Clinic seem to do so effortlessly!. I highly recommend to everyone, whether or not you think you need to give your bones/joints/muscles a 'tune-up' you most probably will benefit from it either way, so give them a chance and I guarantee you won't be disappointed!

Great professional service and friendly and helpful doctors and staff in this well presented and well kept establishment with one of only 3 in the country who practice and are qualified in Osteo and Chiro - definitely recommended from me.

Francis Thomson

ABOUT THE AUTHOR

Since a young age, Dr Trishul Vadi has been deeply passionate about helping people improve their health and wellbeing. This has been the driving force for his obsession with searching for the world for the latest techniques and practices.

Dr Trishul Vadi is one of UK's leading practitioners in drug-free musculo-skeletal treatment and runs AVID Clinic.

In 2006 he received his Bachelors of Osteopathy (BOst) degree from The British School of Osteopathy (London) and in 2012 achieved a Masters in Chiropractic (MChiro) from McTimoney College of Chiropractic in Oxford.

Where to follow Dr Trishul Vadi:

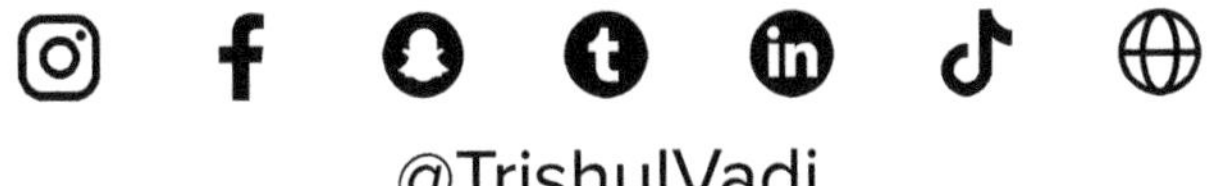

@TrishulVadi

Book a consultation: https://www.avidclinic.co.uk

Trishul Vadi is the leading health care professional in helping your body natural heal itself. He has been interviewed on international television at a Royal Wedding, published articles in professional magazines, and spoken at hundreds of events internationally on his expertise.

NOTES

NOTES

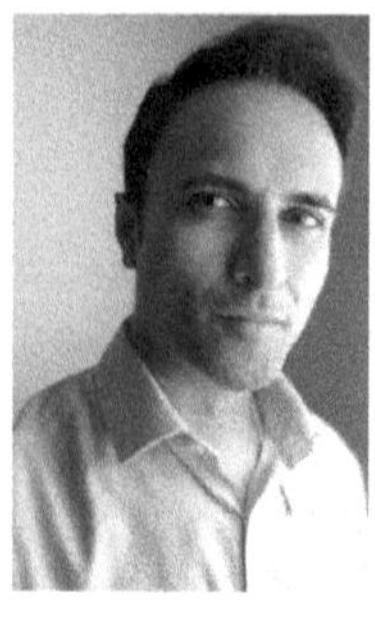

Hi, I'm Dr Trishul Vadi, Clinic Director at AVID Clinic.

I have a big heart to serve you, and as I have limited time in my diary I only see patients by referral.

Therefore if you or someone you know would like to make an appointment with me directly, please let my team know.

Because you have made the awesome life improving decision to get this book in your hands, you will automatically qualify access to my diary.

In the meantime, connect with our community and meet others just like you:
facebook.com/groups/AVIDUniverse

I look forward to meeting you, and serving you directly in person.

Health & Happiness

Dr Trishul Vadi
Osteopath & Doctor of Chiropractic

www.ingramcontent.com/pod-product-compliance
Ingram Content Group UK Ltd.
Pitfield, Milton Keynes, MK11 3LW, UK
UKHW021937190726
13853UKWH00004B/1491

9 798494 188052